Infections in Neutropenic Cancer Patients

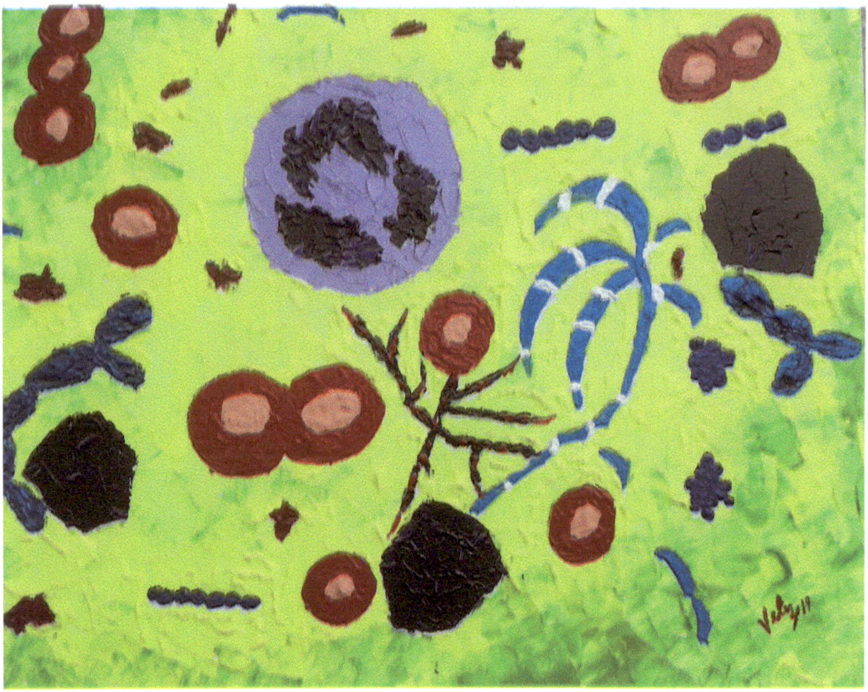

Infections in Neutropenia

Ana Paula Velez • Jorge Lamarche
John N. Greene
Editors

Infections in Neutropenic Cancer Patients

Springer

Editors
Ana Paula Velez
Associate Professor
University of South Florida
Tampa, FL, USA

Jorge Lamarche
James Haley VA Hospital
USF Morsani College of Medicine
Tampa, FL, USA

John N. Greene
Moffitt Cancer Center and Research Institute
USF Morsani College of Medicine
Tampa, FL, USA

ISBN 978-3-030-21858-4 ISBN 978-3-030-21859-1 (eBook)
https://doi.org/10.1007/978-3-030-21859-1

This Springer imprint is published by the registered company Springer Nature Switzerland AG
The registered company address is: Gewerbestrasse 11, 6330 Cham, Switzerland

With love to my parents, my supportive husband, and kids. With all the respect to my colleagues and co-authors, my mentors, and especially to my patients...

Ana Paula Velez

Contents

Central Nervous System Infections in Neutropenic Cancer Patients

Shylah M. Moore-Pardo and Olga Klinkova

Abstract Neutropenic cancer patients are more susceptible to central nervous system (CNS) infections due to impaired host defense mechanisms (Zunt, Neurol Clin 20(1):1–22, 2002). Clinical diagnosis can be challenging due to subtle or atypical presentation or symptoms (Zunt, Neurol Clin 20:1–22, 2002; Lukes et al. Neurology 34(3):269–275, 1984; Schmidt-Hieber et al. Ann Oncol 27(7):1207–1225, 2016). CNS infections typically manifest as four clinical syndromes that may overlap. These are meningitis, encephalitis, brain abscess, and post-surgical neurological infections (Schmidt-Hieber et al. Ann Oncol 27(7):1207–1225, 2016).

Risk factors for CNS infections in this patient population depend on age, type of malignancy, duration of neutropenia, treatment used (type of a transplant, chemotherapy, steroids, immunosuppressant agents, neurosurgical interventions), and environmental exposures.

Keywords Central nervous infections · Bacterial meningitis · Viral meningitis · Non infectious meningitis · Enterovirus meningitis · HSV encephalitis · VZV meningitis · HHV6 encephalitis · JC progressive leukoencephalopathy (PML) · Candida meningitis · Rhomboencephalitis · Brain abscess

Meningitis/Encephalitis

Meningitis is an inflammatory process involving the meninges and is defined by a pleocytosis or abnormal white blood cell count in cerebrospinal fluid (CSF). Encephalitis is a syndrome characterized by inflammation of the brain parenchyma. When these two entities co-exist, meningoencephalitis is diagnosed.

S. M. Moore-Pardo, MD (✉)
Division of Infectious Diseases, Department of Internal Medicine, University of South Florida, Tampa, FL, USA

O. Klinkova, MD
Moffitt Cancer Center, Tampa, FL, USA

A. P. Velez et al. (eds.), *Infections in Neutropenic Cancer Patients*,
https://doi.org/10.1007/978-3-030-21859-1_1

Bacterial meningitis can be classified as community acquired or nosocomial. In neutropenic cancer patients actively receiving chemotherapy, acute bacterial meningitis is a relatively rare diagnosis and the acquisition of infection most commonly occurs through hematogenous spread from other infectious sites or contiguous spread of a pre-existing infection of the head and neck [2]. Patients with prior history of neurosurgical interventions, intraventricular shunts or indwelling vascular devices are at higher risk for bacterial meningitis as well [3, 4]. A true community-acquired meningitis can be seen more frequently in chronically neutropenic patients living in the community.

Noninfectious causes of meningitis that are also important to rule out in cancer patients includes tumor spread (meningeal or parenchymal), vasculitis, and medications (chemotherapy, nonsteroidal anti-inflammatory drugs, sulfa, antithymocyte globulin, intravenous globulin, among others).

Microbiology and Specific Risk Factors

Bacterial Pathogens

Among neutropenic cancer patients, acute bacterial meningitis can be caused by gram positive, gram negative pathogens as well as viruses and atypical bacteria (Table 1). Important gram positive pathogens to consider in this population include *Streptococcus pneumoniae, Staphylococcus aureus,* and coagulase-negative staphylococci [4–6]. Patients undergoing active chemotherapy treatment and with ongoing mucositis are at an increased risk for meningitis caused by *Rothia mucilaginosa* [7, 8] or other gram positive cocci such as Viridans group streptococcus that are a part of normal oral flora. *Corynebacterium jeikeium* meningitis in neutropenic patients has been described in the literature as well [9]. Compared to the general population, *Neisseria meningitides* is a rare cause of meningitis in neutropenic cancer patients [6]. Currently, *Haemophilus influenzae* is rarely seen as a result of Haemophilus influenza type b (Hib) vaccine. *Listeria monocytogenes* is an important cause of meningitis in neonates, older adults, pregnant women, and

Table 1 Meningitis/encephalitis

Bacteria	Virus	Fungi
Streptococcus spp	HSV 1, and HSV 2	*Candida spp*
Neisseria meningitidis	VZV	
Listeria monocytogenes	CMV	
Staphylococcus aureus	EBV	
Coagulase negative staphylococcus (if device in place)	HHV6	
Rothia mucilaginosa	WNV	
Corynebacterium jeikeium	JC virus	
Enterobacteriaceae		
Pseudomonas spp		

immunosuppressed patients (AIDS, chronic steroid use, organ transplants, and those receiving fludarabine chemotherapy) and must be considered in neutropenic patients that live in the community [6, 10, 11].

Gram negative pathogens such as *Enterobacteriaceae* group of organisms and *Pseudomonas aeruginosa* are also an important cause of CNS infection in this population [6].

Viral Pathogens

Enterovirus is by far the most common cause of viral meningitis and should be considered in neutropenic patients that reside in the community [12].

Herpes Simplex Virus-*1, 2* (HSV-1, 2), Varicella Zoster Virus (VZV), cytomegalovirus (CMV), and Epstein Barr Virus (EBV) are potential causative agents of meningoencephalitis in the immunocompromised host. These infections are caused by primary infection or reactivation of latent infection in cancer patients undergoing chemotherapy [1, 13, 14]. VZV is implicated as a cause of not only meningoencephalitis but vasculopathies including vasculitis and cerebro-vascular accidents [15]. CMV spectrum of CNS disease includes meningitis, meningoencephalitis, encephalomyelitis, and radiculopathy [16].

Human Herpes Virus-6 and -8 (HHV-6, −8) frequently reactivate in cancer patients undergoing active chemotherapy. Clinical disease such as encephalitis occurs rarely but should be considered in neutropenic patients with unexplained encephalopathy or other encephalitis symptoms [17, 18]. The most important risk factor for the development of HHV-6 associated encephalitis in this group is a prior history of hematopoietic stem cell transplant (HSCT) with ongoing immunosuppression [17].

Encephalitis due to West Nile Virus (WNV) can be mosquito borne, blood borne, or donor derived in HSCT patients and should be considered in chronically neutropenic patients presenting from the community with encephalitis symptoms.

JC poliomavirus (JC virus) is the cause of progressive multifocal leukoencephalopathy (PML). It is most commonly seen in AIDS patients, but the incidence is increased in cancer patients with certain risk factors [19]. The risk factors that are associated with increased incidence of PML include an underlying diagnosis of lymphoproliferative disease (e.g., B-CLL, Hodgkin's disease), chemotherapy regimens that include purine analogs (e.g., fludarabine, cladribine), rituximab therapy, or low CD4 count [19–21]. Therefore, JC virus should be considered in the differential diagnosis of a neutropenic cancer patient with progressively worsening neurologic symptoms.

Fungal Pathogens

Profound neutropenia and use of total parenteral nutrition have been shown to be risk factors for the development of Candida meningitis in children with malignancies [22]. Other risk factors include preceding fungemia, presence of intra-vascular catheter, or a CNS device. Candida meningitis can also be a result of disseminated candidiasis.

Neutropenic cancer patients are at increased risk for mold infections. *Aspergillus, Zygomycetes*, and *Fusarium spp.* are well-recognized causes of a brain abscess in cancer patients, however, the incidence of an isolated mold meningitis is low [23].

Patients with hematologic malignancies have a higher risk for *Cryptococcus* meningitis [24], however, this is still rare in neutropenic patients.

Clinical Presentation

In those with severely altered immunity and profound neutropenia, symptoms of meningitis/encephalitis can be very subtle, therefore, a high index of suspicion is required to pursue and diagnose these conditions [3, 4]. Based on a prior study by Safdieh et al., only 5% of cancer patients had a classic triad of fever, nuchal rigidity, and altered mental status on presentation [4]. Encephalitis symptoms commonly include altered mentation, confusion, headaches, visual disturbances, focal neurological deficits or seizures.

Laboratory Diagnosis and Imaging

If meningitis or encephalitis is suspected in an immunocompromised host, neuroimaging should be performed as a first step to rule out any focal structural brain abnormalities [3, 25]. Brain CT scan or, if readily available, brain MRI with and without contrast should be performed as soon as possible.

Some MRI findings can highlight clues for specific pathogens. *Listeria monocytogenes* occasionally can cause rhoboencephalitis (inflammation of the brainstem and/or cerebellum). Temporal lobe changes can be seen with HSV, VZV, and HHV6. EBV can cause changes in the caudate nuclei, basal ganglia, thalami, and cortex. CMV as well as HHV6 typically causes ventriculoencephalitis with periventricular enhancement. WNV classically causes changes in the basal ganglia, thalami, and cerebellum, and lastly, JC virus causes multifocal areas of white matter demyelination. (Table 2).

Table 2 Neuroimaging

Organism	Findings
Listeria monocytogenes	Rhomboencephalitis
HSV, VZV, HHV6	Temporal lobe changes
EBV	Caudate nuclei, basal ganglia, thalami, and cortex changes
CMV	Periventricular enhancement
WNV	Basal ganglia, thalami, and cerebellum changes
JC Virus	Multifocal areas of white matter demyelination

Once a space-occupying brain lesion causing brain herniation or a midline shift is ruled out, cerebro-spinal fluid (CSF) analysis should be performed. Blood cultures should be collected as soon as possible and prior to administration of antimicrobial agents if bacterial meningitis is suspected.

During the lumbar puncture, opening pressure should be measured and CSF analysis should be submitted for cell count and differential, cytology, glucose and protein levels. Stains and cultures for bacterial, fungal, and acid-fast organisms should be submitted to the microbiology lab [25, 26]. Currently, most centers have meningitis/encephalitis panels by PCR which is highly sensitive for the detection of common bacterial, viral, and fungal pathogens that cause meningitis and/or encephalitis [27, 28]. However, this test is costly and may not be available in some centers.

CSF pleocytosis is typically seen in cases of acute bacterial meningitis; however, CSF white blood cell count can be either normal or marginally elevated in neutropenic patients [4]. Low CSF glucose and elevated protein are typical findings that are seen in patients with acute bacterial meningitis. The diagnostic yield of Gram-stained smears was shown to be lower in cancer patients compared to the general population [6]. The yield is also lower in patients that have received prior antibiotic therapy [25].

Treatment

If bacterial meningitis is suspected, empiric antimicrobial therapy should be initiated as soon as possible after initial imaging, blood cultures, and CSF studies have been obtained. Antibiotics administration must not be delayed as these infections are associated with high morbidity and mortality [29, 30].

The initial antibiotic regimen in neutropenic cancer patients should cover pathogens seen in the general population with acute bacterial meningitis in addition to methicillin restistant *Staphylococcus aureus* (MRSA) and *Pseudomonas aeruginosa*. Expanded antimicrobial coverage is necessary due to frequently present indwelling devices such as central lines and internalized/externalized CNS shunts. Selected antibiotics must penetrate CNS and achieve an adequate CNS concentration [31]. Third generation cephalosporins such as cefepime or ceftazidime or a carbapenem with anti-pseudomonal activity (such as meropenem or imipenem) plus an anti-MRSA agent are used for the initial therapy [3]. Aztreonam or Ciprofloxacin can be used as an alternative agent in patients with a documented penicillin allergy.

Coverage against *Listeria monocytogenes* should be included with the initial regimen in neutropenic cancer patients that reside in the community and/or have specific risk factors (neutropenia, organ transplant, old age, chronic steroids, pregnant, ingestion of unpasteurized milk or cheese) and clinical presentation concerning for *Listeria* meningitis. Ampicillin or Penicillin G are considered the most active drugs against Listeria; Bactrim or Meropenem can be used as alternatives [3, 25].

Table 3 Treament of viral encephalitis

Virus	Treatment
HSV, VZV	Acyclovir
CMV,HHV6	Gancyclovir/foscarnet
EBV	No specific treatment
WNV	No specific treatment
JC virus	Reversal of immunosuppression if possible

Intravenous acyclovir should be added if there is a concern for HSV encephalitis based on the initial presentation. Gancyclovir or foscarnet can be used to treat CMV or HHV6 encephalitis (Table 3).

Lack of clearance of enterovirus meningitis in lymphoma patients may require the use of intravenous immunoglobulin [32].

Brain Abscess

Patients with neutropenia are at an increased risk for developing a brain abscess [33]. In this patient population, hematogenous spread from other infection sites or a contiguous spread from adjacent structures (face, sinuses, middle ear, teeth) are the most common mechanisms of development of a brain abscess [33]. Cancer patients with history of recent neurosurgeries or CNS catheters such as ventriculo-peritoneal shunts are at increased risk for the development of brain abscess as well [33].

Microbiology

Bacterial Pathogens

The microbiology of the brain abscess differs based on the mechanism of infection acquisition. In patients with neutropenia, gram- negative organisms including Enterobacteriaceae and *Pseudomonas aeruginosa* as well as fungal pathogens are the most important pathogens to be considered [33, 34] (Table 4). Other pathogens such as *Staphylococcus aureus*, streptococci, and anaerobes are also common, especially with hematogenous or contiguous infection spread [33, 35]. If the abscess results from penetrating trauma, *S. aureus*, *S. epidermidis*, Enterobacteriaceae, and Clostridium species may be the culprit [33]. Polymicrobial infections are commonly seen in the general patient population [35] but would be less common in neutropenic patients. Infections with rare bacterial pathogens such as *Nocardia* or *Actinomyces* spp. are likely to be more common in cancer patients especially while on chronic steroids. *Listeria* as an etiology of a brain abscess should be considered in chronically neutropenic patients that reside in the community.

Table 4 Brain abscess

Bacteria	Fungi
Streptococcus spp	*Candida spp*
Staphylococcus aureus	*Aspergillus spp*
Anaerobes	*Mucorales spp*
Enterobacteriaceae	*Scedosporium spp*
Pseudomonas	*Fusarium spp*
Nocardia spp	Dematiaceous fungi

Fungal Pathogens

A high incidence of a fungal brain abscess is reported in neutropenic patients with hematologic malignancies [34]. Most of these infections are acquired through a continuous spread from mold sinusitis causing angioinvasion to the CNS, or from hematogenous spread of the infection from a distal site. Based on the prior studies, *Aspergillus* as well as *Mucorales spp* account for the majority of these infections [34, 36]. Other fungal pathogens such as *Candida spp*, *Scedosporium spp*, *Fusarium spp*, and dematiaceous molds have been reported as well [33, 34, 37] (Table 4).

Clinical Presentation

Patients typically present with headache, fever, focal neurological deficits, seizures, and/or altered mental status. Acute rupture of the abscess into the ventricles may cause meningeal signs. Herniation may occur if intracranial pressure is increased. The presence of coma at the time of presentation is associated with increased mortality.

Laboratory Diagnosis and Imaging

MRI of the brain is the preferred diagnostic modality for the diagnosis of a brain abscess and is considered more sensitive and specific compared to other imaging modalities such as brain CT scan [3, 38]. It typically appears as a single ring enhancing lesion on imaging.

Aspiration of the brain abscess via a stereotactic needle biopsy is frequently needed to establish the causative organism and rule out other potential etiologies such as malignancy [3]. However, when a brain biopsy cannot be obtained or surgery cannot be performed, positive blood cultures and/or identification of an extra neural site of infection may aid the diagnosis. Lumbar puncture might be of low utility in this patient population as it frequently cannot be performed due to concomitant thrombocytopenia. Furthermore, the procedure may increase the risk of herniation when a space-occupying lesion is present.

Treatment

The principles of empiric antimicrobial therapy are similar as described in the "Meningitis/Encephalitis" section. Third generation cephalosporins such as cefepime or ceftazidime or a carbapenem with anti-pseudomonal activity (such as meropenem or imipenem) plus an anti-MRSA agent are used for the initial therapy [3]. Aztreonam or Ciprofloxacin can be used as an alternative agent in patients with a documented penicillin allergy. We recommend addition of anaerobic coverage to the initial antibiotic regimen that could be achieved by addition of metronidazole to a third generation cephalosporin, ciprofloxacin, or Aztreonam.

Coverage for *Listeria monocytogenes* should be included into the initial regimen in neutropenic cancer patients that reside in the community and/or have specific risk factors and clinical presentation concerning for *Listeria* brain abscess. Ampicillin or Penicillin G are considered the most active drugs against Listeria; Bactrim or Meropenem can be used as alternatives [3, 25].

Antifungal therapy either with intravenous voriconazole or liposomal amphotericin B should be included in the initial antimicrobial regimen in the patients with suspected brain abscess [3].

If nocardia is suspected, the addition of trimethoprim/sulfamethoxazole plus imipenem should also be included as part of the initial regimen [39].

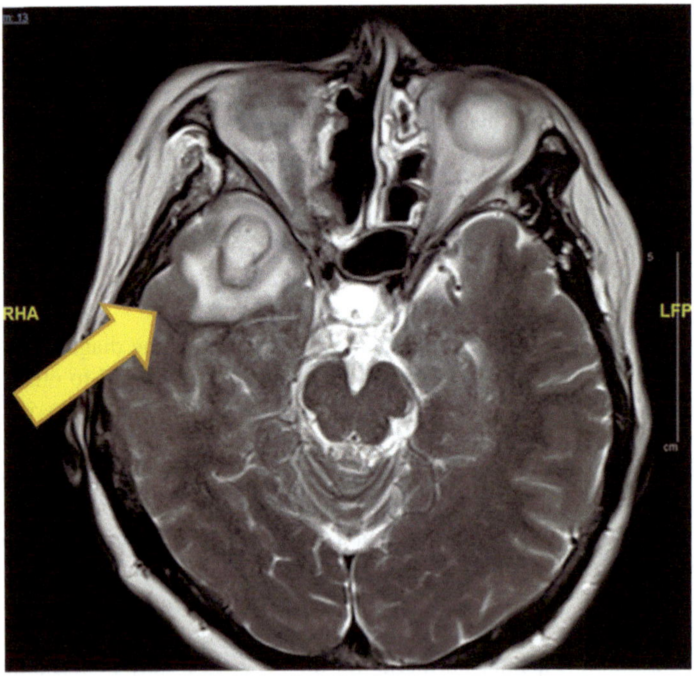

Fig. 1 *Strep intermedius* brain abscess

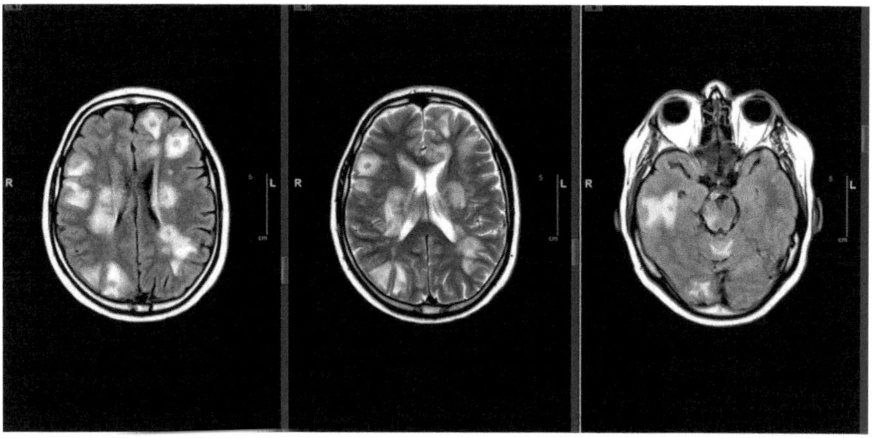

Fig. 2 Nocardia brain abscesses

Once the pathogen has been identified and susceptibilities become available, antimicrobial therapy can be tailored. Broad-spectrum antimicrobial therapy might need to be continued in the patients with negative cultures or when culture data is not available and suspicion for a brain abscess remains high (Figs. 1 and 2).

References

1. Zunt JR. Central nervous system infection during immunosuppression. Neurol Clin. 2002;20(1):1–22.
2. Lukes SA, Posner JB, Nielsen S, Armstrong D. Bacterial infections of the CNS in neutropenic patients. Neurology. 1984;34(3):269–75.
3. Schmidt-Hieber M, Silling G, Schalk E, Heinz W, Panse J, Penack O, et al. CNS infections in patients with hematological disorders (including allogeneic stem-cell transplantation)-Guidelines of the Infectious Diseases Working Party (AGIHO) of the German Society of Hematology and Medical Oncology (DGHO). Ann Oncol. 2016;27(7):1207–25.
4. Safdieh JE, Mead PA, Sepkowitz KA, Kiehn TE, Abrey LE. Bacterial and fungal meningitis in patients with cancer. Neurology. 2008;70(12):943–7.
5. Sommers LM, Hawkins DS. Meningitis in pediatric cancer patients: a review of forty cases from a single institution. Pediatr Infect Dis J. 1999;18(10):902–7.
6. Pomar V, Benito N, Lopez-Contreras J, Coll P, Gurgui M, Domingo P. Characteristics and outcome of spontaneous bacterial meningitis in patients with cancer compared to patients without cancer. Medicine (Baltimore). 2017;96(19):e6899.
7. Gruson D, Hilbert G, Pigneux A, Vargas F, Guisset O, Texier J, et al. Severe infection caused by Stomatococcus mucilaginosus in a neutropenic patient: case report and review of the literature. Hematol Cell Ther. 1998;40(4):167–9.
8. McWhinney PH, Kibbler CC, Gillespie SH, Patel S, Morrison D, Hoffbrand AV, et al. Stomatococcus mucilaginosus: an emerging pathogen in neutropenic patients. Clin Infect Dis. 1992;14(3):641–6.
9. Hoffmann S, Ersgaard H, Justesen T, Friis H. Fatal meningitis with group JK Corynebacterium in a leukopenic patient. Eur J Clin Microbiol. 1983;2(3):213–5.

10. Costerus JM, Brouwer MC, van der Ende A, van de Beek D. Community-acquired bacterial meningitis in adults with cancer or a history of cancer. Neurology. 2016;86(9):860–6.
11. Laguna-Del Estal P, Lledo-Ibanez GM, Rios-Garces R, Pintos-Pascual I. Meningitis due to Listeria monocytogenes in adults. Rev Neurol. 2013;56(1):13–8.
12. Lee BE, Davies HD. Aseptic meningitis. Curr Opin Infect Dis. 2007;20(3):272–7.
13. Graber JJ, Rosenblum MK, DeAngelis LM. Herpes simplex encephalitis in patients with cancer. J Neuro-Oncol. 2011;105(2):415–21.
14. Saito M, Kiyozaki H, Obitsu T, Imoto H, Taniyama Y, Takata O, et al. Herpes simplex virus-1 encephalitis induced by chemoradiotherapy and steroids in an esophageal cancer patient: a case report. BMC Cancer. 2016;16:233.
15. Kleinschmidt-DeMasters BK, Gilden DH. Varicella-Zoster virus infections of the nervous system: clinical and pathologic correlates. Arch Pathol Lab Med. 2001;125(6):770–80.
16. Rafailidis PI, Mourtzoukou EG, Varbobitis IC, Falagas ME. Severe cytomegalovirus infection in apparently immunocompetent patients: a systematic review. Virol J. 2008;5:47.
17. Ongradi J, Ablashi DV, Yoshikawa T, Stercz B, Ogata M. Roseolovirus-associated encephalitis in immunocompetent and immunocompromised individuals. J Neurovirol. 2017;23(1):1–19.
18. Frey JW, Cherabie JN, Assi MA. Human herpesvirus-6 encephalitis following chemotherapy induction for acute myelogenous leukemia. Transpl Infect Dis. 2017;19(6):e12756.
19. Garcia-Suarez J, de Miguel D, Krsnik I, Banas H, Arribas I, Burgaleta C. Changes in the natural history of progressive multifocal leukoencephalopathy in HIV-negative lymphoproliferative disorders: impact of novel therapies. Am J Hematol. 2005;80(4):271–81.
20. Pelosini M, Focosi D, Rita F, Galimberti S, Caracciolo F, Benedetti E, et al. Progressive multifocal leukoencephalopathy: report of three cases in HIV-negative hematological patients and review of literature. Ann Hematol. 2008;87(5):405–12.
21. Yokoyama H, Watanabe T, Maruyama D, Kim SW, Kobayashi Y, Tobinai K. Progressive multifocal leukoencephalopathy in a patient with B-cell lymphoma during rituximab-containing chemotherapy: case report and review of the literature. Int J Hematol. 2008;88(4):443–7.
22. McCullers JA, Vargas SL, Flynn PM, Razzouk BI, Shenep JL. Candidal meningitis in children with cancer. Clin Infect Dis. 2000;31(2):451–7.
23. Antinori S, Corbellino M, Meroni L, Resta F, Sollima S, Tonolini M, et al. Aspergillus meningitis: a rare clinical manifestation of central nervous system aspergillosis. Case report and review of 92 cases. J Infect. 2013;66(3):218–38.
24. Schmalzle SA, Buchwald UK, Gilliam BL, Riedel DJ. Cryptococcus neoformans infection in malignancy. Mycoses. 2016;59(9):542–52.
25. Tunkel AR, Hartman BJ, Kaplan SL, Kaufman BA, Roos KL, Scheld WM, et al. Practice guidelines for the management of bacterial meningitis. Clin Infect Dis. 2004;39(9):1267–84.
26. Dougan C, Ormerod I. A neurologist's approach to the immunosuppressed patient. J Neurol Neurosurg Psychiatry. 2004;75(Suppl 1):i43–9.
27. Liesman RM, Strasburg AP, Heitman AK, Theel ES, Patel R, Binnicker MJ. Evaluation of a commercial multiplex molecular panel for diagnosis of infectious meningitis and encephalitis. J Clin Microbiol. 2018;56(4):e01927–17.
28. Leber AL, Everhart K, Balada-Llasat JM, Cullison J, Daly J, Holt S, et al. Multicenter evaluation of BioFire FilmArray Meningitis/Encephalitis panel for detection of bacteria, viruses, and yeast in cerebrospinal fluid specimens. J Clin Microbiol. 2016;54(9):2251–61.
29. Bodilsen J, Dalager-Pedersen M, Schonheyder HC, Nielsen H. Time to antibiotic therapy and outcome in bacterial meningitis: a Danish population-based cohort study. BMC Infect Dis. 2016;16:392.
30. Miner JR, Heegaard W, Mapes A, Biros M. Presentation, time to antibiotics, and mortality of patients with bacterial meningitis at an urban county medical center. J Emerg Med. 2001;21(4):387–92.
31. Tunkel AR, Hasbun R, Bhimraj A, Byers K, Kaplan SL, Michael Scheld W, et al. 2017 Infectious Diseases Society of America's clinical practice guidelines for healthcare-associated Ventriculitis and meningitis. Clin Infect Dis. 2017;64:701–6 (15 March).

32. Givens P, Velez A, Sandin L, Quilitz R, Greene J. Development of enteroviral aseptic meningitis after rituximab treatment of non-hodgkin lymphoma. Infect Dis Clin Pract. 2012;20:291–3.
33. Brouwer MC, Tunkel AR, McKhann GM 2nd, van de Beek D. Brain abscess. N Engl J Med. 2014;371(5):447–56.
34. Economides MP, Ballester LY, Kumar VA, Jiang Y, Tarrand J, Prieto V, et al. Invasive mold infections of the central nervous system in patients with hematologic cancer or stem cell transplantation (2000–2016): uncommon, with improved survival but still deadly often. J Infect. 2017;75(6):572–80.
35. Brook I. Microbiology and treatment of brain abscess. J Clin Neurosci. 2017;38:8–12.
36. Pagano L, Caira M, Falcucci P, Fianchi L. Fungal CNS infections in patients with hematologic malignancy. Expert Rev Anti-Infect Ther. 2005;3(5):775–85.
37. Garcia RR, Min Z, Narasimhan S, Bhanot N. Fusarium brain abscess: case report and literature review. Mycoses. 2015;58(1):22–6.
38. Shih RY, Koeller KK. Bacterial, fungal, and parasitic infections of the central nervous system: radiologic-pathologic correlation and historical perspectives. Radiographics. 2015;35(4):1141–69.
39. Kim S, Lee KL, Lee DM, Jeong JH, Moon SM, Seo YH, et al. Nocardia brain abscess in an immunocompetent patient. Infect Chemother. 2014;46(1):45–9.

Head and Neck Infections

Ana Paula Velez, John N. Greene, and Jorge A. Lamarche

Abstract The head and neck have several compartments with very rich blood and nerve supply. Organisms from the oral cavity and skin can gain access to the vital structures of the head and neck causing severe infection. The infection can spread rapidly to vital locations causing life threathening complications. Prompt diagnosis and therapy are essential especially in neutropenic patients.

In this chapter we will review the most common infections of the head and neck seen in neutropenic patients.

Keywords Malignant otitis · Periorbital cellulitis · Necrotizing gingivitis · Vincent's angina · Herpetic gingivostomatitis · Submandibular space infections · Ludwing's angina · Lateral pharyngeal space infection · Retropharyngeal and prevertebral space infections

Malignant Otitis Externa

Malignant otitis externa is an infection of the external canal with the potential spread to soft tissues, cartilage and bone. The most common bacteria isolated include *pseudomonas, staphylococcus aureus, aspergillus* spp, *klebsiella oxytoca,*

A. P. Velez, MD, FACP (✉)
Associate Professor, University of South Florida, Tampa, FL, USA
e-mail: ana.velez@moffitt.org

J. N. Greene, MD, FACP
USF Morsani College of Medicine, Moffitt Cancer Center and Research Institute, Tampa, FL, USA

Department of Infectious Diseases, University of South Florida, Tampa, FL, USA

J. A. Lamarche, MD
Nephrology Department, University of South Florida Morsani College of Medicine, Tampa, FL, USA

James Haley VA Hospital, Tampa, FL, USA

A. P. Velez et al. (eds.), *Infections in Neutropenic Cancer Patients*,
https://doi.org/10.1007/978-3-030-21859-1_2

proteus mirabilis, burkholderia cepacia, and candida parapsilosis. The infection has been classically reported in elderly diabetic patients, AIDS patients, and patients with other types of immunosuppression [1–6].

The clinical manifestations include otorrhea, and otalgia mainly nocturnal with severe pain radiated to the temporomandibular joint.

In neutropenic patients, the infection can be secondary to molds and it is usually severe and potentially lethal causing osteomyelitis of the base of the skull, VII cranial nerve palsy, and brain abscess [7–9].

The diagnosis is usually clinical and microbiological. Radiological studies such as computed tomography (CT), and magnetic resonance imaging (MRI) can complement the diagnosis, but does not always correlate with the clinical course [10].

It is paramount to obtain gram stain and cultures from the ear discharge for microbiologic diagnosis and therapy. These cultures should include bacteria as well as fungus.

The treatment is debridement and antibiotics directed to the organisms isolated. Empiric antibiotics pending the culture results should include agents to cover *pseudomonas* and *staphylococcus aureus* (including methicillin resistant). Ideal choices include vancomycin plus cefepime, ceftazidime, piperacillin-tazobactam, or carbapenem such as imipenem, meropenem or doripenem. Quinolones such as ciprofloxacin and levofloxacin are widely used as prophylaxis in this population, therefore concerns for pseudomonas resistant malignant otitis remains a concern. Quinolones may still be an acceptable option provided that the pseudomonas isolated in the ear culture is still suceptible. If *aspergillus spp.* is isolated, the ideal choice is voriconazole, alternatively lipid amphotericin can be used [11].

Periorbital Cellulitis

Periorbital cellulitis is an infection of the tissues around the bony orbit. The most common cause of periorbital cellulitis in non-neutropenic patients include *H. influenza, staphylococcus aureus,* and *streptococcus spp.* [12]. In neutropenic patient molds such as *mucorales spp*, *aspergillus spp*, and *fusarium spp* are also very important pathogens. In such cases the infection usually spread from the sinuses to the periorbital tissues [13–15].

Periorbital cellulitis is further divided into preseptal or postseptal (orbital) depending on the area of infection. Preseptal cellulitis is an infection of the eyelid and the skin anterior to the orbital septum (Fig. 1). Postseptal (orbital cellulitis) is an infection posterior to the orbital septum. It involves the muscles and fat of the orbit. Postseptal cellulitis is a potential lethal infection. The infection may originate after local skin trauma (scratch, insect bite) with skin flora causing the infection or from direct spread from the sinuses to the orbit [16]. The latter is the most common cause of orbital cellulitis in neutropenic patients.

Clinical symptoms include edema, erythema and superficial pain. Pain with ocular movement, proptosis, diplopia and opthalmoplegia may be a sign of post septal cellulitis. If a mold infection is present, a nasal or palate necrotic eschar can be seen

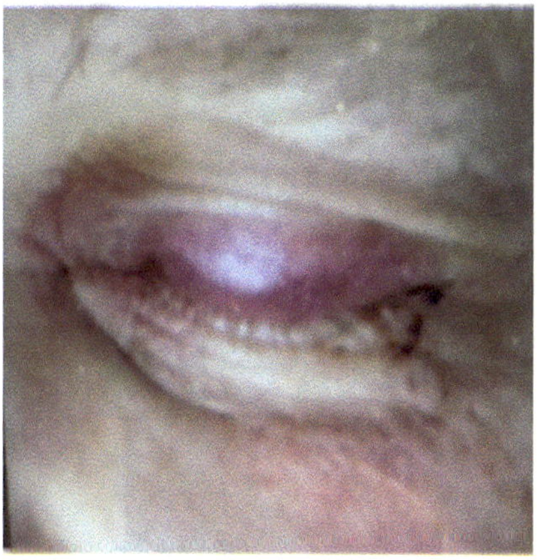

Fig. 1 Patient with preseptal cellulitis

on physical examination. Mold infections can rapidly cause angioinvasion spreading to the brain causing vascular thrombosis and tissue infarction [15].

The diagnosis of orbital cellulitis is based on clinical symptoms and physical examination. Radiological imaging such as CT of the orbit and sinuses are indicated in this population to rule out concomitant sinusitis.

If sinusitis is seen, an otorhinolaryngologist (ENT) specialist should be consulted for deeper evaluation and debridement of the sinuses. Mucosal samples should be sent to microbiology for gram stain, bacterial and fungal cultures. If deep tissue is obtained, the tissue should also be sent for special fungal stains.

Empiric therapy with vancomycin plus piperacillin tazobactam, cefepime, ceftazidime, or carbapenem such as imipenem, meropenem or doripenem, plus an antifungal such as lipid amphotericin should be started pending microbiological information. Combination of antifungal therapy with an azole or an echinocandin can be attempted in severe immunosuppressed patients but its use is still controversial [15]. Once the microbiological information is obtained, the antimicrobial therapy can be de-escalated to target the isolated pathogen.

Oral Mucosa Infections and Necrotizing Gingivitis

Mucotoxic chemotherapy can cause extensive inflammation to the oral mucosa leading to mucositis, which can be complicated by periodontal infections, gingivitis, and gum ulcers [17–19].

The oral flora of the immunocompromised patients change as a result of the chemotherapy and prophylactic antibiotics. Bacteria, other than the usual oral flora, such as pseudomonas can colonize the mucosa causing or complicating preexisting necrotic gum ulcer or gingivitis [17, 20] (Fig. 2). Other important pathogens that can spread from the mucosa to the blood stream in neutropenic patients with mucositis include *Streptococcus mitis*, *Fusobacterium spp*, *Klebsiella*, *E coli*, *Enterobacter spp* and *Stomatococcus spp*. [21, 22]

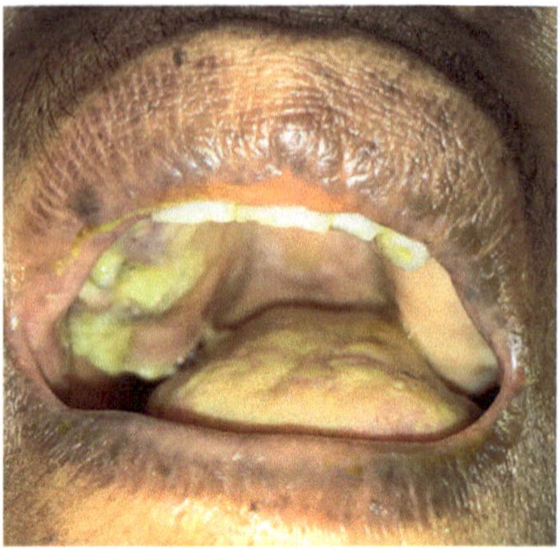

Fig. 2 Patient with pseudomonas necrotizing gingivitis

The latter can also be associated with gum or buccal mucosa ulcers that can be complicated by Vincent's Angina or trench mouth. This infection is a rapidly progressive necrotizing gingivostomatitis visualized as necrotic tissue with a grayish-white pseudomembrane [23]. *Fusobacterium spp* and other anaerobes can spread further causing deep neck infections discussed later in this chapter.

Candida spp can cause thrush in neutropenic patients, particularly in the absence of antifungal prophylaxis. Thrush is visualized as white creamy plaques in the tongue, palate and buccal mucosa. The plaques are usually associated with satellite lesions. Erythematous plaques without membranes and angular cheilosis can also be caused by candida infection. The differential diagnosis of thrush is hairy tongue. Hairy tongue is caused by abnormal desquamation of the filiform papillae resulting from several factors [24].

Herpetic gingivostomatitis is caused by herpes simplex virus (HSV) type 1 and rarely type 2. In the setting of hematological malignancy, reactivation may occur in up to 60% of the cases and in up to 80% in bone marrow transplant recipients that are not on prophylaxis. Given immunosuppression, the neutropenia and the thrombocytopenia, the clinical manifestations of HSV may not be classical. Ulcers with irregular or serpentiginous borders or extensive hemorrhagic lesions can be seen in place of the typical cluster vesicles (Fig. 3). Given the atypical presentation, HSV lesions may be confused with trauma. Alternatively, HSV reactivation may also occur from minor trauma caused by oral –gastric and endotracheal tubes. Occasionally, the lesions may progress despite of acyclovir, famciclovir, or valacyclovir. In such cases, the diagnosis of HSV acyclovir resistant virus needs to be considered and the therapy may have to be changed to foscarnet [25, 26].

It is important to perform a complete oral examination to detect any buccal or gingival ulcer. If an ulcer is detected, swab for gram stain, bacterial, fungal cultures and HSV PCR should also be obtained.

The empiric treatment of necrotizing gingivitis in neutropenic patients should be with piperacillin tazobactam or cefepime plus metronidazole or ceftazidime plus metronidazole, meropenem, imipenem, or doripenem pending cultures. Clindamycin can be an alternative to metronidazole. If HSV is isolated or suspected, famciclovir

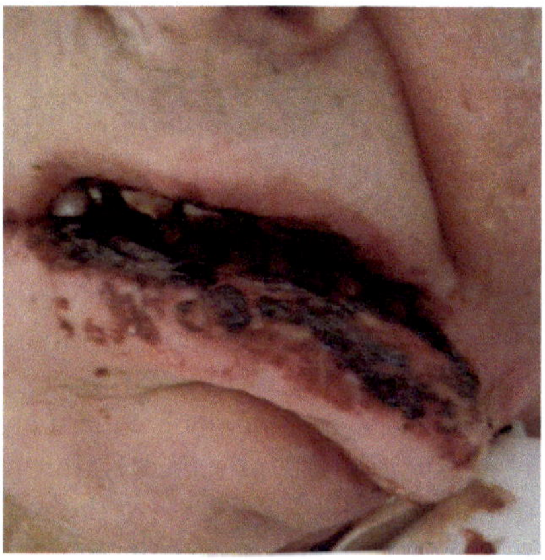

Fig. 3 Patient with hemorrhagic HSV

or valacyclovir should be added. Further therapy can be de-escalated to target the specific organism once the results of the cultures are available.

Cervicofacial Space Infections

Submandibular Space Infections

The submandibular space infections are also known as Ludwing's angina. This infection is caused by cellulitis of the bilateral sublingual, and submental space. The culprit is usually an infection of the second or third mandibular molar, but non odontogenic infections or unknown etiology can also cause it [27].

On physical exam, the patient has drooling, dysphagia, stridor, and fever. The mouth is usually open and the tongue is edematous displaced against the palate. An area of induration and with crepitus may be felt under the submandibular area. The patient usually lean forward to maximize the diameter of the airway [28]. If untreated, the infection can progress to lymphangitis, submandibular face cellulitis with progression to necrotizing fasciitis and mediastinitis.

The disease is commonly polymicrobial including *peptostreptococcus spp*, *fusobacterium spp*, *prevotella spp*, *Staphylococcus aureus*, and *Pseudomonas spp*. Other enteric gram negatives are also important pathogens in neutropenic patients [28].

The treatment is with systemic antibiotics discussed below. If rapid progression of the infection or worsening edema is seen, protection of the airway should be ensured. Intubation including tracheostomy before stridor or obvious airway compromise is seen must be preformed. Systemic antibiotics such as Vancomycin, plus piperacillin tazobactam, or cefepime plus metronidazole, or ceftazidime plus metronidazole, or metronidazole, meropenem, imipenem, or doripenem should be started as soon as possible. Clindamycin can be an alternative to metronidazole.

If fluctuance is appreciated or clinical deterioration is seen in 36–48 hours, needle aspiration or debridement should be done [28].

Infections of the Lateral Pharyngeal Space

This compartment is further divided into anterior and posterior compartments by the styloid process. The posterior compartment and the cranial nerves IX to XII are within the posterior compartmental space. Infections of the lateral pharyngeal space carry high morbidity and mortality because they can spread to the carotid sheath leading to hematogenous dissemination. Dental infections, tonsillar abscess (quinsy abscess or postanginal sepsis), otitis, mastoiditis or parotitis are usually the infections of the lateral pharyngeal space.

Clinical symptoms include trismus, edema below the angle of the mandibula, fever, and sepsis. Unfortunately, this infection can spread rapidly especially in neutropenic patients, and involve the retropharyngeal space and the mediastinum. In these cases, surgery is an emergency.

Complications of the lateral pharyngeal space include suppurative internal jugular thrombophlebitis or postanginal sepsis also known as Lemierre's syndrome (Fig. 4). Most cases are caused by *Fusobacterium necrophorum.* Other potential involved bacteria include Bacteriodes, *Eikenella*, Streptococcus, peptostreptococcus, Porphyromonas, Prevotella, Proteus, meticillin-sensitive *Staphylococcus aureus,* and meticillin-resistant *Staphylococcus aureus* [29].

Lemierre's syndrome develops from lymphatic spread of infection. Trismus is usually absent and the patient may present only with fever of unknown origin with systemic toxicity. Unilateral sore throat may be present but not universally. Dyspnea may develop as the infection involves the epiglottis and the larynx.

Suppurative jugular thrombophlebitis is a feared vascular complication. Trismus may be minimal or absent, vocal cord palsy or cranial nerve involvement may be

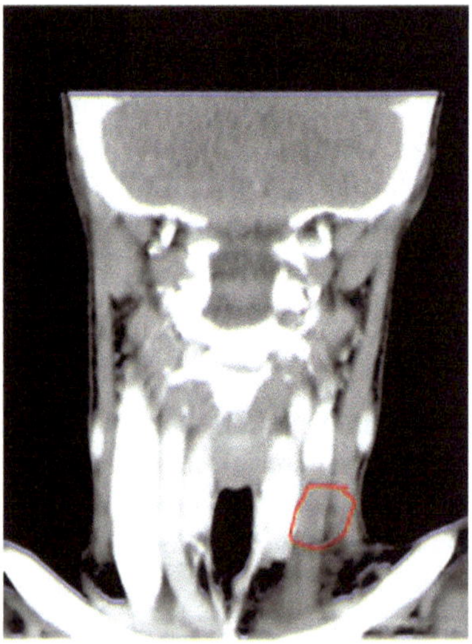

Fig. 4 CT of the neck demonstrates left jugular vein thrombosis (red circle) in a patient with Lemierre's syndrome

present. On physical examination, small area of edema may be palpated behind the sternocleidomastoid muscle [29]. Metastatic abscess to the lung, bones, and joints may develop. If retrograde dissemination occurs, meningitis or brain abscess may develop.

The treatment of the lateral pharyngeal space infections is with the same systemic antibiotics discussed for infections of the submandibular space. CT scan may be useful to localize the infection and determine the presence of local suppuration. If local suppuration is seen, needle aspiration may be considered or required [28].

In patients with acute leukemia tonsilar or oral sweet's syndrome may present similarly to the infections discussed above. Biopsy is crucial to make the diagnosis. Steroids are indispensable to prevent airway obstruction [30].

Infections of the Retropharyngeal and Prevertebral Space

Infections of this space are rare but life threatening (danger space) (Fig. 5) since the infection can spread directly into the anterior and posterior portion of the upper mediastinum. Necrotizing mediastinitis may develop with rupture into the pleural cavity causing empyema. Pericarditis with infected pericardial effusions and even tamponade may also complicate the picture.

Prompt diagnosis and debridement are the mainstays of treatment. Systemic antibiotics as discussed for submandibular infections are also indicated [28].

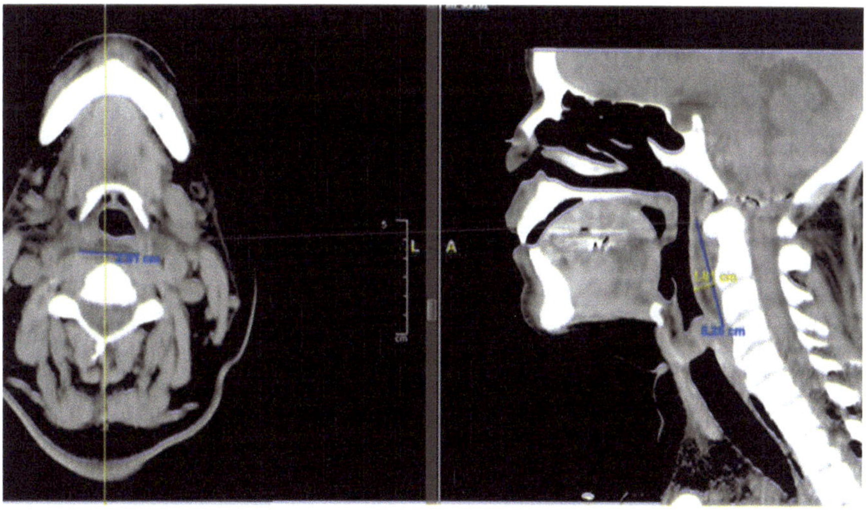

Fig. 5 CT of the neck of a patient with C3-C4 prevertebral abscess

Key Points

Disease	Organisms	Treatment
Malignant otitis externa	*Pseudomonas, Staphylococcus aureus, Aspergillus, Klebsiella oxytoca, Proteus mirabilis, Burkholderia cepacia*, and *Candida parapsilosis*	Vancomycin plus one of the following: cefepime, ceftazidime, piperacillin-tazobactam, or carbapenem. Vancomycin plus quinolone if the organism is proven to be sensitive.
Periorbital cellulitis	*H. influenza, staphylococcus aureus, streptococcus spp, mocorales, aspergillus spp*, and *fusarium spp*	Vancomycin plus one of the following: piperacillin tazobactam cefepime, ceftazidime, or carbapenem plus an antifungal such as lipid amphotericin pending microbiological information. ENT consult
Mucosal infections and necrotizing gingivitis	*Streptococcus mitis spp, stomatococcus spp, fusobacterium spp*, and other anaerobes, *candida spp* and HSV, *Pseudomonas*, MDR GNR	Piperacillin tazobactam, or cefepime plus metronidazole, or ceftazidime plus metronidazole, or carbapenem plus fluconazole. Clindamycin can be an alternative to metronidazole. If HSV is isolated or suspected, famciclovir or valacyclovir.
Neck space infections	*Peptostreptococcus spp., fusobacterium spp., prevotella spp. Staphylococcus aureus, Psudomonas spp.* and other enteric gram negatives	Vancomycin, plus one of the following: piperacillin tazobactam, or cefepime plus metronidazole, or ceftazidime plus metronidazole, or meropenem, or imipenem, or doripenem. Clindamycin can be an alternative to metronidazole. Steroids to prevent airway obstruction. ENT evaluation

References

1. Bayardelle P, Jolivet-Granger M, Larochelle D. Staphylococcal malignant external otitis. Can Med Assoc J. 1982;126(2):155–6.
2. Coser PL, Stamm AE, Lobo RC, Pinto JA. Malignant external otitis in infants. Laryngoscope. 1980;90(2):312–6.
3. Cunningham M, Yu VL, Turner J, Curtin H. Necrotizing otitis externa due to Aspergillus in an immunocompetent patient. Arch Otolaryngol Head Neck Surg. 1988;114(5):554–6.
4. Munoz A, Martinez-Chamorro E. Necrotizing external otitis caused by Aspergillus fumigatus: computed tomography and high resolution magnetic resonance imaging in an AIDS patient. J Laryngol Otol. 1998;112(1):98–102.
5. Phillips P, Bryce G, Shepherd J, Mintz D. Invasive external otitis caused by Aspergillus. Rev Infect Dis. 1990;12(2):277–81.
6. Rubin J, Yu VL. Malignant external otitis: insights into pathogenesis, clinical manifestations, diagnosis, and therapy. Am J Med. 1988;85(3):391–8.
7. Davis JC, Gates GA, Lerner C, Davis MG Jr, Mader JT, Dinesman A. Adjuvant hyperbaric oxygen in malignant external otitis. Arch Otolaryngol Head Neck Surg. 1992;118(1):89–93.
8. Sreepada GS, Kwartler JA. Skull base osteomyelitis secondary to malignant otitis externa. Curr Opin Otolaryngol Head Neck Surg. 2003;11(5):316–23.

9. Finer G, Greenberg D, Leibovitz E, Leiberman A, Shelef I, Kapelushnik J. Conservative treatment of malignant (invasive) external otitis caused by Aspergillus flavus with oral itraconazole solution in a neutropenic patient. Scand J Infect Dis. 2002;34(3):227–9.
10. Al-Noury K, Lotfy A. Computed tomography and magnetic resonance imaging findings before and after treatment of patients with malignant external otitis. Eur Arch Otorhinolaryngol. 2011;268(12):1727–34.
11. Patterson TF, Thompson GR 3rd, Denning DW, Fishman JA, Hadley S, Herbrecht R, et al. Executive summary: practice guidelines for the diagnosis and management of Aspergillosis: 2016 update by the Infectious Diseases Society of America. Clin Infect Dis. 2016;63(4):433–42.
12. Ambati BK, Ambati J, Azar N, Stratton L, Schmidt EV. Periorbital and orbital cellulitis before and after the advent of Haemophilus influenzae type B vaccination. Ophthalmology. 2000;107(8):1450–3.
13. Rutar T, Cockerham KP. Periorbital zygomycosis (mucormycosis) treated with posaconazole. Am J Ophthalmol. 2006;142(1):187–8.
14. Cho HJ, Jang MS, Hong SD, Chung SK, Kim HY, Dhong HJ. Prognostic factors for survival in patients with acute invasive fungal rhinosinusitis. Am J Rhinol Allergy. 2015;29(1):48–53.
15. Davoudi S, Kumar VA, Jiang Y, Kupferman M, Kontoyiannis DP. Invasive mould sinusitis in patients with haematological malignancies: a 10 year single-centre study. J Antimicrob Chemother. 2015;70(10):2899–905.
16. Ganesh A, Venugopalan P. Preseptal orbital cellulitis following oral trauma. J Pediatr Ophthalmol Strabismus. 2000;37(5):315–7.
17. Kamasaki Y, Satoh K, Nishiguchi M, Hoshino T, Fujiwara T. Acute oral complications in a pediatric patient with acute lymphoid leukemia. Pediatr Int. 2016;58(6):484–7.
18. Peterson DE, Bensadoun RJ, Roila F. Management of oral and gastrointestinal mucositis: ESMO clinical practice guidelines. Ann Oncol. 2011;22(Suppl 6):vi78–84.
19. Villa A, Sonis ST. Mucositis: pathobiology and management. Curr Opin Oncol. 2015;27(3):159–64.
20. Sampson MM, Nanjappa S, Greene JN. Mucositis and oral infections secondary to gram negative rods in patients with prolonged neutropenia. IDCases. 2017;9:101–3.
21. Terhes G, Piukovics K, Urban E, Nagy E. Four cases of bacteraemia caused by fusobacterium nucleatum in febrile, neutropenic patients. J Med Microbiol. 2011;60.(Pt 7:1046–9.
22. Kitten T, Munro CL, Zollar NQ, Lee SP, Patel RD. Oral streptococcal bacteremia in hospitalized patients: taxonomic identification and clinical characterization. J Clin Microbiol. 2012;50(3):1039–42.
23. Pistacchio E. Plaut-Vincent's angina. Infez Med. 1999;7(4):260–3.
24. Gurvits GE, Tan A. Black hairy tongue syndrome. World J Gastroenterol. 2014;20(31):10845–50.
25. Iino T, Gondo H, Ohno Y, Minagawa H, Iwasaki H, Maruyama T, et al. Successful foscarnet therapy for mucocutaneous infection with herpes simplex virus in a recipient after unrelated bone marrow transplantation. Bone Marrow Transplant. 1996;18(6):1185–8.
26. Darville JM, Ley BE, Roome AP, Foot AB. Acyclovir-resistant herpes simplex virus infections in a bone marrow transplant population. Bone Marrow Transplant. 1998;22(6):587–9.
27. Botha A, Jacobs F, Postma C. Retrospective analysis of etiology and comorbid diseases associated with Ludwig's Angina. Ann Maxillofac Surg. 2015;5(2):168–73.
28. Chow AW. Life-threatening infections of the head and neck. Infect Dis Clin North Am. 1992;14(5):991–1002.
29. Kuppalli K, Livorsi D, Talati NJ, Osborn M. Lemierre's syndrome due to fusobacterium necrophorum. Lancet Infect Dis. 2012;12(10):808–15.
30. Qiao J, Wang Y, Bai J, Wu Y, Fang H. Concurrence of Sweet's syndrome, pathergy phenomenon and erythema nodosum-like lesions. An Bras Dermatol. 2015;90(2):237–9.

Respiratory Infections

Olga Klinkova

Abstract Pneumonia is defined as the presence of a new pulmonary infiltrate on radiologic imaging in the patient with appropriate clinical symptoms such as fever, cough, production of purulent sputum, shortness of breath and/or hypoxia, in the absence of pulmonary edema [1, 2].

Keywords Pneumonia in neutropenic cancer patients · Community acquired viruses · Invasive fungal infection · Diffuse alveolar hemorrhage (DAH) · Cryptogenic organizing pneumonia (COP) · Consolidation pneumonia · Nodular and/or cavitary infiltrates · "Halo" sign · Reverse "halo" sign · Scattered nodules · Viral pneumonia · Rhinosinusitis

Pneumonia/Pulmonary Infiltrates

Introduction

Pneumonia is defined as the presence of a new pulmonary infiltrate on radiologic imaging in the patient with appropriate clinical symptoms such as fever, cough, production of purulent sputum, shortness of breath and/or hypoxia, in the absence of pulmonary edema [1, 2].

Absolute as well as functional neutropenia is the most important risk factor for development of pneumonia in cancer patients [3]. Duration of neutropenia is another important factor to consider as the etiology of pneumonia may differ in patients with prolonged (>15 days) neutropenia. Additionally, in patients undergoing hematopoietic stem cell transplant (HCT), time lapsed after transplant, antimicrobial prophylaxis

O. Klinkova, MD (✉)
Moffitt Cancer Center, Tampa, FL, USA
e-mail: olga.klinkova@moffitt.org

A. P. Velez et al. (eds.), *Infections in Neutropenic Cancer Patients*,
https://doi.org/10.1007/978-3-030-21859-1_3

and intensity of immunosuppression should be considered, as these variables predict the development of certain pneumonia types in this unique patient population.

Microbiology

Bacterial Pathogens

Similar to the general patient population, pneumonia in neutropenic cancer patients can be classified based on the mode of acquisition into community-acquired pneumonia (CAP), hospital-acquired pneumonia (HAP), and ventilator-associated pneumonia (VAP).

CAP is defined as the type of pneumonia that develops in patients who have not been recently hospitalized. A true CAP is infrequently observed in neutropenic patients. CAP may be considered in patients with chronic prolonged neutropenia residing in the community as well as in neutropenic patients with newly diagnosed hematologic malignancies starting active chemotherapy. The most frequent pathogen causing CAP in cancer patients is *Streptococcus pneumoniae* [3, 4]. Other bacterial pathogens in neutropenic cancer patients causing CAP include *Haemophilus influenzae*, *Staphylococcus aureus* and *Pseudomonas aeruginosa.* Atypical pathogens such as *Legionella spp.*, *Chlamydophila pneumoniae* and *Mycoplasma pneumoniae* should be included into the differential diagnosis as well.

HAP is defined as a pneumonia that is not present at the time of admission and instead occurs 48 hours or more after admission, whereas VAP is defined as pneumonia occurring 48 hours or more after intubation [1].

HAP and VAP are caused by a broad spectrum of pathogens with gram-negative bacilli being the most prevalent in the neutropenic cancer patient population [5–7]. The organisms that should be always considered include *Pseudomonas aeruginosa*, *Escherichia coli*, *Klebsiella pneumoniae*, *Enterobacter spp.*, *Serratia spp.* and *Acinetobacter spp.* [5, 7]. *Staphylococcus aureus* is the most common gram-positive pathogen causing HAP/VAP. *Streptococcus pneumoniae*, *Haemophilus influenzae* could also be encountered, especially in patients with minimal or no recent exposure to antibiotics or the hospital environment [3]. Isolation of certain gram-positive organisms from the blood or sputum samples, such as *Viridans group streptococcus*, *Enterococcus spp.*, *Bacillus spp.*, should be interpreted with caution as they are rarely implicated in the development of pneumonia. In such cases alternative source/pathogens need to be considered [7]. Table 1 illustrates the list of the most commonly encountered bacterial pathogens in neutropenic patients.

The majority of neutropenic cancer patients are at risk for the development of multidrug resistant pathogens due to antimicrobial prophylaxis use, extensive exposure to broad-spectrum antibiotics as well as the nosocomial environment [8, 9]. Forty to eighty percent of *Staphylococcus aureus* isolates are methicillin-resistant [9]. The most important mechanisms of gram-negative organism resistance include the production of various beta-lactamases such as Ambler class C (AmpC) beta-lactamases and extended-spectrum beta-lactamases (ESBL). The emergence of carbapenem- resistant

Table 1 Etiologic agents of pneumonia in neutropenic patients

Bacterial	Viral	Fungal
Gram-positive	Influenza A/B virus	Aspergillus spp.
Streptococcus pneumoniae	Parainfluenza virus	Zygomycetes
Staphylococcus aureus	Human metapneumovirus virus	Fusarium spp.
Beta-hemolytic Streptococcus	RSV	Scedosporium spp.
Streptococcus Viridans	Adenovirus	Dark-walled fungi
Rhodococcus equi	CMV	Histoplasma capsulatum
Gram-negative	VZV	Coccidioides immitis
Haemophilus influenzae	HSV	Blastomyces dermatididis
Moraxella Catarrhalis	HHV-6	Pneumocystis jiroveci
Pseudomonas Aeruginosa		
Escherichia Coli		
Klebsiella Pneumoniae		
Enterobacter cloacae		
Serratia spp.		
Proteus spp.		
Acınetobacter baumanii complex		
Stenotrophomonas maltophila		
Burkholderia spp.		
Atypical bacteria		
Legionella spp.		
Chlamydophila pneumoniae		
Mycoplasma pleumoniae		
Mycobacteria		
Mycobacterium tuberculosis		
Nontuberculous mycobacerium		
Other pathogens		
Nocardia spp.		
Actynomyces spp.		

Enterobacteriaceae (CRE) is concerning. It has been associated with a delay in necessary appropriate antibiotic therapy and high mortality in cancer patients [10].

Viral Pathogens

Community-acquired viruses such as enterovirus/rhinovirus, influenza, respiratory syncytial virus (RSV) and other community-acquired viruses are commonly seen in neutropenic patients [3, 7]. In patients post HSCT and other severely immunocompromised patients, cytomegalovirus (CMV), varicella zoster virus (VZV) and, less commonly, HHV-6 should be considered as etiologic agents along with other viruses [7, 11] (Table 1).

Fungal Pathogens

In patients with profound (ANC < 500) and/or prolonged duration of neutropenia (>10 days), in addition to the above mentioned etiologies, fungal pathogens should be strongly considered [12]. *Aspergillus fumigatus* is the most common fungal pathogen causing pneumonia in this patient population. *Aspergillus spp.*, *Zygomycetes*, *Fusarium spp.*, *Pseudaalesheria boydii*, and dark-walled fungi are other potential etiologies that cause fungal pneumonia [3, 12, 13]. Endemic fungal pneumonias caused by *Histoplasma capsulatum*, *Coccidioides immitis* and *Blastomyces dermatididis* can occasionally occur, but are less common in neutropenic patients [3, 12].

Neutropenic patients with associated CD4 + cell depletion not receiving appropriate prophylaxis are at high risk for *Pneumocystis jiroveci* pneumonia [14, 15]. Examples include patients with acute lymphoblastic leukemia, those receiving CD4 + cell-depleting chemotherapy or chronic corticosteroids (equivalent of 20 mg/day prednisone for more than 1 month).

Other Pathogens

Rhodococcus, Actynomyces spp., *Nocardia spp.* and *Mycobacterium spp.* should be also considered [7, 16] in the etiology of pneumonia in neutropenic patients, especially with a subacute presentation.

Clinical Manifestations

Fever, increased production of purulent sputum, dyspnea, and decrease in oxygenation along with the findings of a new infiltrate are signs of pneumonia. In neutropenic patients, the symptoms can be rather subtle or atypical. Pleuritic chest pain and hemoptysis may be present as well.

Differential Diagnosis

The differential diagnosis of pulmonary infiltrates in a neutropenic patient is broad. Other etiologies that should be considered include acute respiratory distress syndrome (ARDS), transfusion related lung injury (TRALI), diffuse alveolar hemorrhage(DAH), drug and radiation toxicity or pneumonitis, cryptogenic organizing pneumonia (COP), cardiogenic and non-cardiogenic pulmonary edema from capillary leak and the underlying malignancy [2, 17].

Diagnosis and Radiologic Findings

Chest radiograph has a low sensitivity for early detection of pulmonary infiltrates in febrile neutropenic patients [17–19].This is especially true given the broad differential diagnosis discussed above Therefore, chest computed tomography (CT) is now considered the standard imaging procedure for diagnosing pneumonia in this patient

Table 2 Key radiologic features of pneumonia caused by different fungal agents

Fungal organism	Radiologic appearance
Aspergillus spp.	Few or single segmental nodular consolidations (diameter > 1–2 cm) Few or single ground glass opacities with lobular distributions Infiltrates mostly peripherally located Nodular infiltrate with surrounded by ground glass infiltrate "Halo" sign
Zygomycetes	Nodular consolidations (diameter > 2 cm), mostly peripherally located Ground glass surrounded by an area of consolidation Reverse "Halo" sign. With or without Pleural effusion
Fusarium spp.	Scattered nodular consolidations (multiple (>2), average diameter < 1 cm)
Scedosporium spp.	Scattered nodular consolidations (multiple (>2), diameter 1–2 cm)

population. The number, characteristics and distribution of the infiltrates can help with the differential diagnosis and guide with a choice of empiric antimicrobial therapy (Table 2).

Consolidation pneumonia can be caused by bacterial pathogens such as s. aureus, pseudomonas, and enterobacteriaceae. Legionella can cause ground glass or consolidation pneumonia (Fig. 1). Diffuse bilateral infiltrates and bilateral ground-glass attenuation should raise clinical suspicion for atypical pathogens, viral (Fig. 2), or PJ pneumonia (Fig. 3) or a non-infectious etiology [18] (Fig. 4).

Nodular and/or cavitary infiltrates indicate the possibility of invasive fungal infection (IFI), especially in patients with prolonged duration of neutropenia (>10 days). The "halo" sign is defined as a nodule (typically >1 cm) surrounded by a perimeter of ground-glass opacity representing hemorrhage [20] (Fig. 5) This sign is commonly seen in patients with invasive pulmonary aspergillosis (IPA) [17, 21]. The reverse "halo" sign, defined as a focal area of ground glass attenuation surrounded by consolidation (Fig. 6) is more frequently observed with zygomycosis [22, 23]. *Fusarium* pulmonary infections are typically characterized by the presence of multiple small (<1 cm) scattered nodules [23].

To establish a microbiologic diagnosis, sputum and blood cultures should be obtained. Streptococcus pneumoniae, Legionella urinary antigens and the respiratory viral panel PCR panel can assist with rapid diagnosis if positive. When IPA is suspected, it is strongly recommended to obtain serum galactomannan (GM) in patients with hematologic malignancies [18, 20].

Unless the etiology of pneumonia was established in an expedited manner using non-invasive rapid diagnostic testing or culture method as indicated above, bronchoscopy with bronchoalveolar lavage (BAL) for cultures should be strongly considered in a febrile neutropenic patient with new pulmonary infiltrates [18, 24, 25]. Active bleeding or severe hypoxia might not allow early bronchoscopy, but it is generally considered a safe procedure in this patient population [24]. BAL sample should be sent for "standard", fungal, mycobacterial, nocardia, Legionella cultures, respiratory viral panel and cytology. Based on prior studies, measurement of BAL GM may offer even higher sensitivity comparing to the performance of blood GM assays for the diagnosis of invasive fungal pneumonia [12, 13].

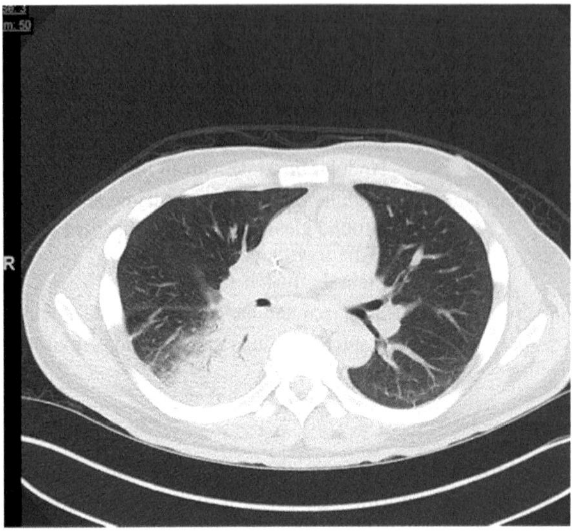

Fig. 1 Chest CT of a patient with Legionella pneumonia

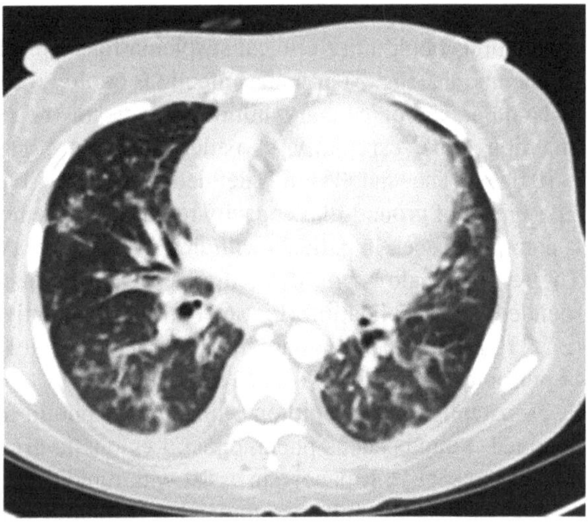

Fig. 2 Chest CT of a patient with RSV pneumonia

Trans bronchial biopsy is rarely used in this patient population due to severe thrombocytopenia and risk of complications such as a life-threatening bleeding. CT-guided percutaneous lung biopsy can be considered for the patient with large peripheral lesions if the diagnosis is expected to change medical management and the benefits of the procedure outweigh its risks.

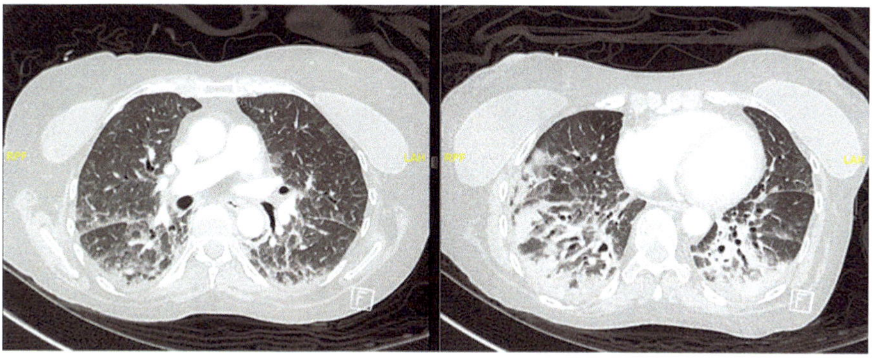

Fig. 3 Chest CT of a patient with PJP pneumonia

Fig. 4 Chest CT of a patient with DAH

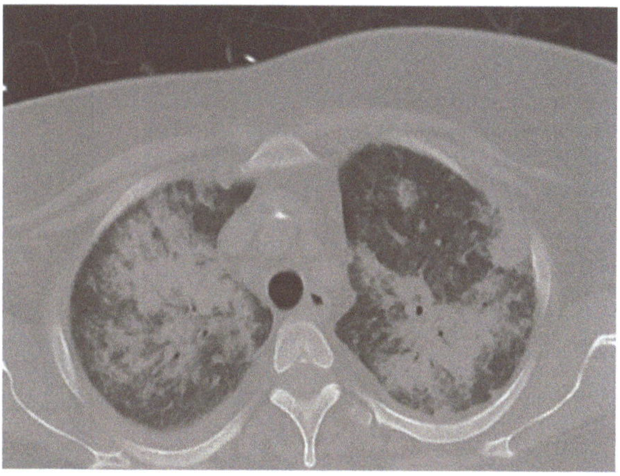

Treatment

Antibiotic therapy should be initiated as soon as the blood and sputum cultures are obtained, but should not be held if there is a delay in obtaining a diagnostic work-up.

Initial empiric antibiotic regimens of a newly diagnosed pneumonia in a febrile neutropenic patient should include broad-spectrum antibiotic agents to cover Pseudomonas and S. aureus (including MRSA) [26]. Patients at risk for multidrug-resistant pathogens or with a prior history of such, as well as patients at high risk for mortality at the time of presentation (septic shock or pneumonia requiring ventilator support) should be prescribed two anti-pseudomonal agents from different classes until further information from the cultures is available [1]. Beta-lactam antibiotics with anti-pseudomonal coverage include cefepime, ceftazidime, piperacillin-tazobactam, or a carbapenem with anti-pseudomonal activity such as meropenem or imipenem. Aztreonam can be used as an alternative agent in patients with a documented penicillin allergy. A second anti-pseudomonal agent can be either an

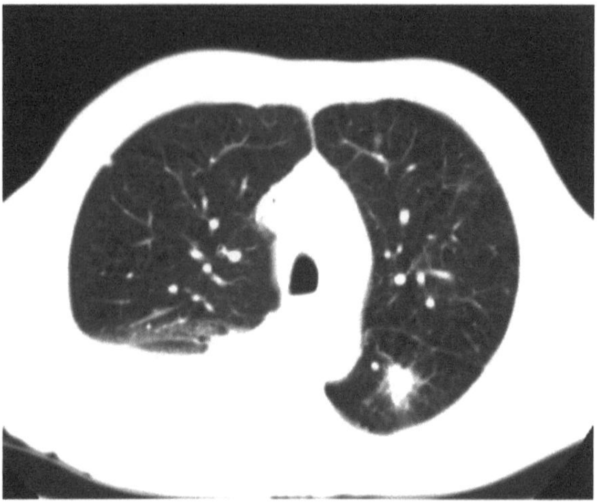

Fig. 5 CT chest with the halo sign

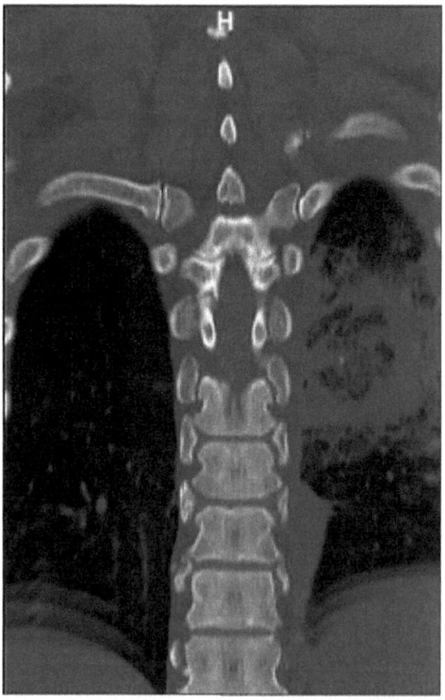

Fig. 6 Chest CT with the reverse halo sign

aminoglycoside or a fluoroquinolone; however, neither of these antibiotics should be used as sole agents. Aminoglycoside monotherapy for the treatment of pneumonia is not recommended due to poor lung penetration and alveolar concentration, prompting higher antibiotic dosing that potentially can lead to nephro- and ototoxicity [1, 27]. Fluoroquinolone monotherapy is discouraged due to the increasing rate of resistance to this particular antibiotic class. Agents with MRSA coverage, vancomycin or linezolid, should also be included into the initial treatment regimen of pneumonia.

In neutropenic cancer patients with a true community-acquired pneumonia or an early hospital acquired pneumonia, an agent with coverage against atypical pathogens such as *Legionella spp.*, *Mycoplasma spp.* and *Chlamydophila pneumoniae* should be included into the regimen. Fluoroquinolones, doxycycline or azithromycin should be a part of the regimen in such clinical scenarios [28].

Anti-fungal therapy should be initiated in neutropenic patients with high suspicion for invasive fungal pneumonia on radiographic testing or in the patients that do not appropriately respond to the initial antibiotic regimen, [3, 18]. Voriconazole or liposomal amphotericin B remains the preferred first-line regimen. In patients with suspected mucormycosis, liposomal amphotericin B is the preferred first-line agent for the initial therapy. Primary monotherapy with echinocandins is not recommended due to low treatment response rates in patients with IPA [13, 20]. Combination regimens with two different anti-fungal agents are typically reserved as a salvage therapy in the treatment of IPA and mucormycosis [3, 13, 20].

In patients with suspected PJ pneumonia, first line therapy with high-dose trimethoprim–sulfamethoxazole (TMP/SMX) should be initiated [18, 29]. In patients with allergic reactions or contraindications to TMP/SMX, a combination therapy with clindamycin plus primaquine may be considered as an alternative [18, 29]. Routine adjunctive therapy with steroids in non-HIV patients with the diagnosis of PJ pneumonia is not recommended [18, 29, 30].

Treatment of viral pneumonia is based on the etiologic agent. CMV pneumonia is treated with intravenous gancyclovir or foscarnet with a combination of intravenous immunoglobulin or CMV-specific immunoglobulin [18, 31, 32]. Due to the side effect of pancytopenia, ganciclovir is generally contraindicated in the settings of severe neutropenia or a pre-engraftment phase of HSCT [31, 32]. For the treatment of influenza A and B infections, neuraminidase inhibitors, such as oseltamivir, zanamivir, or peramivir are recommended [31]. RSV pneumonia is typically treated with aerosolized, oral or intravenous ribavirin [31, 33, 34]. Addition of intravenous immunoglobulin may further reduce mortality in this patient population [35]. In high-risk patients with severe human metapneumovirus (hMPV) pneumonia, ribavirin treatment may be used as well but the use of this agent remains controversial [31, 36]. For the treatment of parainfluenza virus (PIV), the use of ribavirin has been described in the literature; albeit without any evidence of reduced mortality [37]. Treatment with interferon Alpha-2b for severe PIV pneumonia may be another promising therapeutic option that needs to be studied further [38].

Rhinosinusitis

Introduction

Rhinosinusitis is defined as inflammation of the nasal cavity and paranasal sinuses [39]. Neutropenic patients with cancer are at increased risk for unusual microorganisms as a cause of rhinosinusitis as well as development of invasive or complicated disease.

Microbiology

In a healthy (not immune-compromised) host, community-acquired viruses such as rhinovirus, influenza and parainfluenza are responsible for the development of sinusitis [40] and should be considered in neutropenic patients with this condition as well. When a bacterial infection occurs, causative organisms to consider in this patient population are *Pseudomonas aeruginosa*, *Staphylococcus aureus*, *Streptococcus pneumoniae*, *Haemophilus influenzae*, and *Moraxella catarrhalis* [41, 42]. Oral anaerobic flora such as *Prevotella spp.*, *Fusobacterium spp.* and *Peptostreptococcus spp.* are implicated as well, especially in chronic sinusitis [40]. Fungal/mold pathogen such as *Aspergillus spp.*, *mucorales*, *Fusarium spp.*, and dematiaceous fungi are the causes of invasive fungal sinusitis, commonly seen in patients with prolonged neutropenia [43].

Clinical Manifestations

Purulent nasal drainage, nasal congestion, facial pain and pressure are the most common signs of acute sinusitis [39, 41]. Fever might be present in some of the patients. In complicated sinusitis, the infection might spread beyond the paranasal sinuses and nasal cavity. In such cases, oculo-orbital and CNS symptoms such as periorbital edema, erythema, vision changes, cranial nerve palsy, meningismus or focal neurologic symptoms might occur. The presence of necrotic eschars in the oral or nasal cavities should raise a high suspicion for invasive fungal process.

Diagnosis

In febrile neutropenic patient with acute sinusitis, CT sinuses is typically the first diagnostic modality and can evaluate the extent of sinus involvement including possible fungal bony erosion or orbital invasion [44]. (Fig. 7).MRI sinuses could be used as an alternative imaging technique or if intracranial or cavernous sinus involvement is suspected. Early direct endoscopic visualization of the nasal mucosa by an otolaryngologist should be pursued [45]. Endoscopic biopsies and cultures of the affected tissues are typically positive to establish the diagnosis.

Nasopharyngeal swab for a respiratory viral panel aids in the diagnosis of uncomplicated viral sinusitis. Nasal swab cultures are not recommended due to their poor reliability.

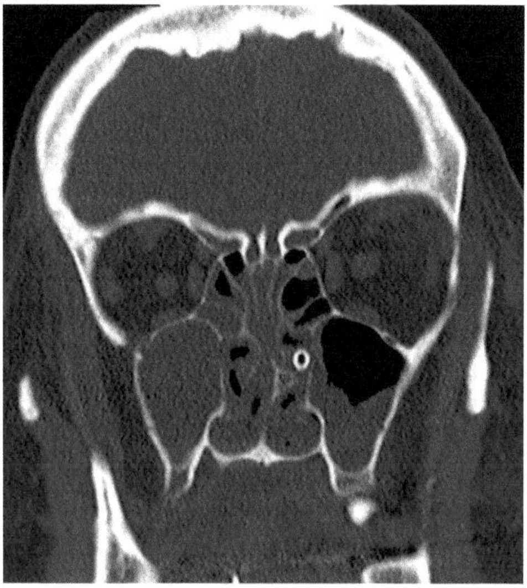

Fig. 7 CT sinuses of a patient with mold sinusitis

Treatment

Febrile neutropenic patients with diagnosis of acute bacterial sinusitis should receive broad-spectrum antibiotics with anti-pseudomonal activity until culture results become available. These antibiotic options include cefepime, ceftazidime, piperacillin-tazobactam or an anti-pseudomonal carbapenem such as meropenem, imipenem or doripenem. The decision to include anti-MRSA agent, such as vancomycin or linezolid, should be based on patient-specific risk factors and the severity of the illness.

When invasive fungal sinusitis is suspected in a patient with prolonged neutropenia, treatment should not be delayed. Voriconazole, isavuconazole or liposomal amphotericin B are first-line options. In patients with high suspicion for invasive mucormycosis, liposomal amphotericin B is considered to be the drug of choice for initial therapy. Early surgical debridement by an otolaryngologist must be considered in such cases.

References

1. Kalil AC, et al. Management of adults with hospital-acquired and ventilator-associated pneumonia: 2016 clinical practice guidelines by the Infectious Diseases Society of America and the American Thoracic Society. Clin Infect Dis. 2016;63(5):e61–e111.
2. Vehreschild JJ. Pneumonia and lung infiltrates in neutropenic patients: many stones unturned. Ann Am Thorac Soc. 2013;10(5):493–5.
3. Evans SE, Ost DE. Pneumonia in the neutropenic cancer patient. Curr Opin Pulm Med. 2015;21(3):260–71.

4. Sousa D, et al. Community-acquired pneumonia in immunocompromised older patients: incidence, causative organisms and outcome. Clin Microbiol Infect. 2013;19(2):187–92.
5. American Thoracic Society, Infectious Diseases Society of America. Guidelines for the management of adults with hospital-acquired, ventilator-associated, and healthcare-associated pneumonia. Am J Respir Crit Care Med. 2005;171(4):388–416.
6. Lossos IS, et al. Bacterial pneumonia in recipients of bone marrow transplantation. A five-year prospective study. Transplantation. 1995;60(7):672–8.
7. Rolston KV. The spectrum of pulmonary infections in cancer patients. Curr Opin Oncol. 2001;13(4):218–23.
8. Perez F, Adachi J, Bonomo RA. Antibiotic-resistant gram-negative bacterial infections in patients with cancer. Clin Infect Dis. 2014;59(Suppl 5):S335–9.
9. Rapoport B, et al. The emerging problem of bacterial resistance in cancer patients; proceedings of a workshop held by MASCC "Neutropenia, Infection and Myelosuppression" Study Group during the MASCC annual meeting held in Berlin on 27–29 June 2013. Support Care Cancer. 2016;24(7):2819–26.
10. Satlin MJ, et al. Emergence of carbapenem-resistant Enterobacteriaceae as causes of bloodstream infections in patients with hematologic malignancies. Leuk Lymphoma. 2013;54(4):799–806.
11. Konoplev S, et al. Cytomegalovirus pneumonia in adult autologous blood and marrow transplant recipients. Bone Marrow Transplant. 2001;27(8):877–81.
12. Young AY, Leiva Juarez MM, Evans SE. Fungal pneumonia in patients with hematologic malignancy and hematopoietic stem cell transplantation. Clin Chest Med. 2017;38(3):479–91.
13. Mulanovich VE, Kontoyiannis DP. Fungal pneumonia in patients with hematologic malignancies: current approach and management. Curr Opin Infect Dis. 2011;24(4):323–32.
14. Souza JP, et al. High rates of pneumocystis carinii pneumonia in allogeneic blood and marrow transplant recipients receiving dapsone prophylaxis. Clin Infect Dis. 1999;29(6):1467–71.
15. Yale SH, Limper AH. Pneumocystis carinii pneumonia in patients without acquired immunodeficiency syndrome: associated illness and prior corticosteroid therapy. Mayo Clin Proc. 1996;71(1):5–13.
16. Henkle E, Winthrop KL. Nontuberculous mycobacteria infections in immunosuppressed hosts. Clin Chest Med. 2015;36(1):91–9.
17. Maschmeyer G. Pneumonia in febrile neutropenic patients: radiologic diagnosis. Curr Opin Oncol. 2001;13(4):229–35.
18. Maschmeyer G, et al. Diagnosis and antimicrobial therapy of lung infiltrates in febrile neutropenic patients (allogeneic SCT excluded): updated guidelines of the infectious diseases working party (AGIHO) of the German Society of Hematology and Medical Oncology (DGHO). Ann Oncol. 2015;26(1):21–33.
19. Maschmeyer G, et al. Diagnosis and antimicrobial therapy of lung infiltrates in febrile neutropenic patients: guidelines of the infectious diseases working party of the German Society of Haematology and Oncology. Eur J Cancer. 2009;45(14):2462–72.
20. Patterson TF, et al. Practice guidelines for the diagnosis and management of aspergillosis: 2016 update by the Infectious Diseases Society of America. Clin Infect Dis. 2016;63(4):e1–e60.
21. Satish Kumar Bajaj BT. Respiratory infections in immunocompromised patients: lung findings using chest computed tomography. Radiol Infect Dis. 2017;4:29–37.
22. Wahba H, et al. Reversed halo sign in invasive pulmonary fungal infections. Clin Infect Dis. 2008;46(11):1733–7.
23. Farooq A, Alrabaa S, Quilitz R, Yacoub A, Maroon ME, Fulp W, Sandin R, Greene JN. Comparison of clinical and radiological features of aspergillus, zygomycosis, and fusarium pneumonia in neutropenic patients. Infect Dis Clin Pract. 2014;22(5):288–93.
24. Hohenadel IA, et al. Role of bronchoalveolar lavage in immunocompromised patients with pneumonia treated with a broad spectrum antibiotic and antifungal regimen. Thorax. 2001;56(2):115–20.

25. Kuehnhardt D, et al. Therapeutic implication of BAL in patients with neutropenia. Ann Hematol. 2009;88(12):1249–56.
26. Freifeld AG, et al. Clinical practice guideline for the use of antimicrobial agents in neutropenic patients with cancer: 2010 update by the infectious diseases society of america. Clin Infect Dis. 2011;52(4):e56–93.
27. Carcas AJ, et al. Tobramycin penetration into epithelial lining fluid of patients with pneumonia. Clin Pharmacol Ther. 1999;65(3):245–50.
28. Mandell LA, et al. Infectious Diseases Society of America/American Thoracic Society consensus guidelines on the management of community-acquired pneumonia in adults. Clin Infect Dis. 2007;44(Suppl 2):S27–72.
29. Maschmeyer G, et al. ECIL guidelines for treatment of pneumocystis jirovecii pneumonia in non-HIV-infected haematology patients. J Antimicrob Chemother. 2016;71(9):2405–13.
30. Lemiale V, et al. Adjunctive steroid in HIV-negative patients with severe pneumocystis pneumonia. Respir Res. 2013;14:87.
31. Vakil E, Evans SE. Viral pneumonia in patients with hematologic malignancy or hematopoietic stem cell transplantation. Clin Chest Med. 2017;38(1):97–111.
32. Marchesi F, et al. Cytomegalovirus infection in hematologic malignancy settings other than the allogeneic transplant. Hematol Oncol. 2018;36(2):381–91.
33. Khanna N, et al. Respiratory syncytial virus infection in patients with hematological diseases: single-center study and review of the literature. Clin Infect Dis. 2008;46(3):402–12.
34. Weigt SS, et al. Respiratory viral infections in hematopoietic stem cell and solid organ transplant recipients. Semin Respir Crit Care Med. 2011;32(4):471–93.
35. Torres HA, et al. Characteristics and outcome of respiratory syncytial virus infection in patients with leukemia. Haematologica. 2007;92(9):1216–23.
36. Waghmare A, Englund JA, Boeckh M. How I treat respiratory viral infections in the setting of intensive chemotherapy or hematopoietic cell transplantation. Blood. 2016;127(22):2682–92.
37. Chemaly RF, et al. The characteristics and outcomes of parainfluenza virus infections in 200 patients with leukemia or recipients of hematopoietic stem cell transplantation. Blood. 2012;119(12):2738–45; quiz 2969.
38. Marinez J, Vincent AL, Sandin RL, Greene JN. Interferon Alfa-2b as a successful treatment for parainfluenza virus pneumonia in a non-hodgkin lymphoma patient. Infect Dis Clin Pract. 2008;16(3):187–9.
39. Rosenfeld RM. CLINICAL PRACTICE. Acute sinusitis in adults. N Engl J Med. 2016;375(10):962–70.
40. Brook I. Microbiology of sinusitis. Proc Am Thorac Soc. 2011;8(1):90–100.
41. Rosenfeld RM, et al. Clinical practice guideline (update): adult sinusitis. Otolaryngol Head Neck Surg. 2015;152(2 Suppl):S1–S39.
42. Ito CJ, Jackson RS, Castro-Borobio M, Nanjappa S, Klinkova O, Phommachanh V, Keeler JA, Greene JN, Padhya TA, Tabor MH. Microbiology of acute rhinosinusitis in immunosuppressed patients. Infect Dis Clin Pract. 2017;25:260–3.
43. Davoudi S, et al. Invasive mould sinusitis in patients with haematological malignancies: a 10 year single-centre study. J Antimicrob Chemother. 2015;70(10):2899–905.
44. DelGaudio JM, et al. Computed tomographic findings in patients with invasive fungal sinusitis. Arch Otolaryngol Head Neck Surg. 2003;129(2):236–40.
45. DelGaudio JM, Clemson LA. An early detection protocol for invasive fungal sinusitis in neutropenic patients successfully reduces extent of disease at presentation and long term morbidity. Laryngoscope. 2009;119(1):180–3.

Gastrointestinal and Genitourinary Infections

Ana Paula Velez, John N. Greene, and Jorge Lamarche

Abstract Gastrointestinal infections in neutropenic patients are common especially in the setting of mucotoxic chemotherapy. In this setting common enteric pathogens can easily gain access to the bloodstream and cause bacteremia and severe sepsis. Additionally, other gastrointestinal infections commonly seen in immunocompetent patients such as *clostridium difficile* colitis can often complicate the clinical picture in neutropenic patients given the broad use of antibiotics.

Genitourinary infections in neutropenic patients occur as a complication of indwelling foley catheters, mucosal inflammation and anatomical abnormalities of the genitourinary tract. Although the pathogenesis is similar to the immunocompetent population, the infections are more frequent and severe in neutropenic patients.

In this chapter, we will discuss the most common type of gastrointestinal and genitourinary tract infections in neutropenic patients.

Keywords Candida esophagitis · HSV esophagitis · CMV esophagitis · Neutropenic colitis · Typhlitis · *Clostridium difficile* colitis · Proctitis · Diverticulitis · Hepatitis B and C virus · Hemorrhagic viral cystitis

Esophagitis

Neutropenic patients are particularly predisposed to develop infectious esophagitis given the chemotherapy induced mucositis, radiation therapy, immunosuppression, steroid use and prophylactic antibiotics. In this section, we will review the most

A. P. Velez, MD, FACP (✉)
Associate Professor, University of South Florida, Tampa, FL, USA
e-mail: ana.velez@moffitt.org

J. N. Greene, MD, FACP
USF Morsani College of Medicine, Moffitt Cancer Center and Research Institute, Tampa, FL, USA

J. Lamarche, MD
USF Morsani College of Medicine, James Haley VA Hospital, Tampa, FL, USA

A. P. Velez et al. (eds.), *Infections in Neutropenic Cancer Patients*,
https://doi.org/10.1007/978-3-030-21859-1_4

common cause of esophagitis including candida, herpes simplex (HSV) and cytomegalovirus (CMV). Other causes of esophagitis such as pill esophagitis, radiation and eosinophilic esophagitis, as well as other non-infections causes of esophagitis are not within the scope of this book.

Candida Esophagitis

Candia albicans is the most common type of *candida spp* that cause candida esophagitis but other type of *candida spp.* such as *c. glabrata, c. kruseii, and c. tropicalis* can also cause esophagitis in neutropenic patients [1].

Clinical symptoms of candida esophagitis include odynophagia and retrosternal pain. Oral or soft palate thrush may be a clue on physical examination, but is not always present [2].

The diagnosis of candida esophagitis is by endoscopy. White plaques are seen attached to the esophageal mucosa (Fig. 1). Mucosal samples demonstrate yeast and pseudohyphae. Cultures reveal *candida spp.*

The treatment of candida esophagitis is with empiric systemic antifungals based on the above symptoms. If the symptoms do not improve in 72 hours, endoscopy should be performed to rule out other causes of esophagitis [3].

The use of topical antifungal agents to treat candida esophagitis should be avoided. Systemic fluconazole is the agent of choice. Fluconazole resistant candida esophagitis should be suspected if the symptoms do not improve, especially patients who have been on prophylactic fluconazole, voriconazole, posaconazole, or isavuconazole. In such cases micafungin or amphotericin should be considered. The recommended length of treatment is 14–21 days [4].

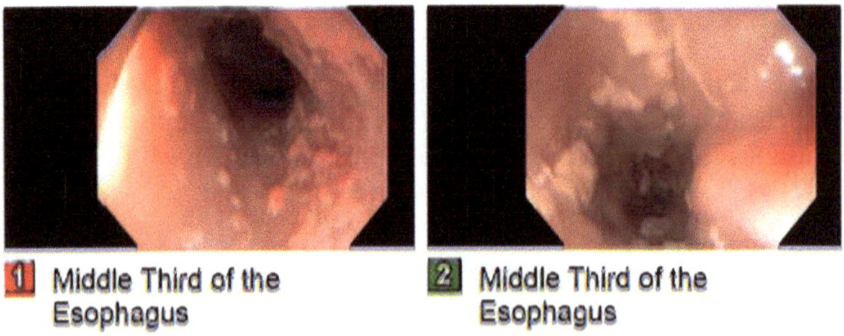

Fig. 1 Endoscopic picture demonstrating candida esophagitis

Herpes Simplex Virus Esophagitis

The majority of Herpes Virus Simplex (HSV) esophagitis are due to HSV1, but HSV2 can also be isolated [5]. Patients usually complaint of dysphagia, odynophagia, retrosternal pain with or without fever [6]. In addition, intractable hiccups has also been described [7].

On physical examination, oral vesicles or ulcers may be present, but not always as the infection may be deeper in the esophagus.

The diagnosis of HSV esophagitis relies on endoscopic observation of small coalescent ulcers less than 2 cm in diameter (Fig. 2). Biopsy of the suspicious lesions should be taken to confirm the diagnosis. Histopathology of the tissue demonstrates multinucleated giant cells. The tissue should also be sent for HSV stains and culture.

Qualitative PCR from the tissue samples can be used, but this technique is highly sensitive and can be associated with asymptomatic viral shedding that does not necessarily correlates with clinical findings especially if no ulcers are visualized [8].

The treatment of HSV esophagitis in neutropenic patients should be for 14–21 days. Famciclovir or valacyclovir can be used. If the patient is not able to tolerate medications by mouth, IV acyclovir can be prescribed.

Acyclovir by mouth is often used, but may not be as convenient as oral famciclovir or valacyclovir because the absorption is less predictable and it has to be taken several times a day.

If the patients do not respond to initial therapy, HSV resistant virus should be suspected. In such cases, the initial therapy may have to be changed to foscarnet. If biopsy samples are available, they should be tested for thymidine kinase gene mutation. This mutation is associated with HSV resistance to valacyclovir and famciclovir [9].

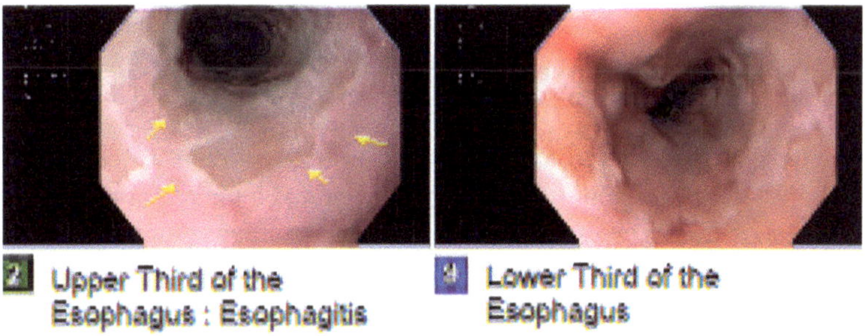

Fig. 2 Endoscopic picture of HSV esophagitis

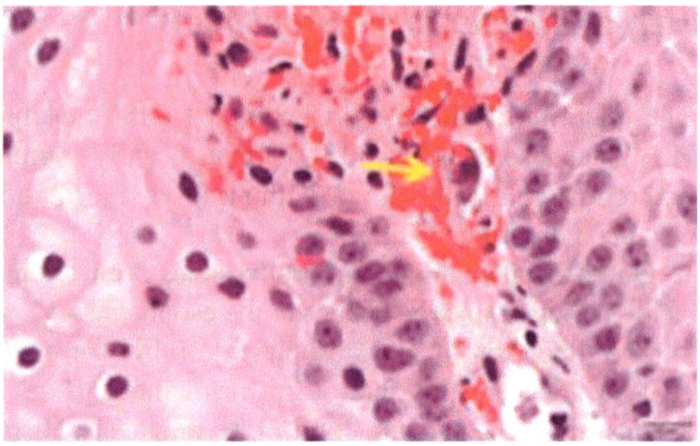

Fig. 3 Typical intranuclear and intracytoplasmic inclusions with the characteristic cytomegalic cells

Cytomegalovirus Esophagitis

Cytomegalovirus (CMV) esophagitis is the second most common type of CMV infection after CMV colitis in immunosuppressed patients. In cancer patients, risk factors include radiation therapy, chemotherapy, and immunosuppression therapy. Clinical manifestations are similar to HSV and candida esophagitis including, odynophagia, dysphagia, retrosternal chest pain, nausea and vomiting [10].

The diagnosis of CMV esophagitis is by endoscopic evaluation of the lesions and biopsy with tissue samples assessed for histopathology. The lesions are typically linear or shallow erosions. Tissue biopsy reveals the typical intranuclear and intracytoplasmic inclusions with the characteristic cytomegalic cells (Fig. 3). CMV PCR in blood may not useful because it does not always correlate with organ disease [11, 12].

The treatment for CMV esophagitis is ganciclovir, or its prodrug valganciclovir. Other options particularly for CMV resistant virus include foscarnet or cidofovir. The last 2 options are only reserved for patients who are intolerant or resistant to ganciclovir given their potential nephrotoxicity [13–15].

Colitis, Proctitis and Diverticulitis

Neutropenic patients are particularly predisposed to develop different causes of colitis. Prophylactic antibiotics, chemotherapy, and radiation therapy can be associated with mucositis and enteritis. Enteric flora and previous colonizing bacteria can cause local infection and translocate to the blood stream.

Neutropenic colitis known as typhlitis, and *clostridium difficile* colitis are the most common type of colitis in neutropenic patients and will be reviewed here. Other infectious causes of colitis such as CMV, adenovirus, rotavirus, norovirus, and parasitc colitis are not within the scope of this chapter.

Neutropenic Colitis

Typhlitis is a life threatening enterocolitis that occurs mainly in neutropenic patients. The pathogenesis is poorly understood, but it is believed that chemotherapy induced mucosal injury, and motility dysfunction with bacterial overgrowth causing secondary bacterial infection may play a role. The most common affected area is the cecum followed by the ascending colon and the terminal ileum. It has been postulated that the distensibility of the cecum and limited blood supply may facilitate the bacterial overgrowth [16–18].

Typhlitis is usually a polymicrobial infection with several bacteria involved including *Klebsiella spp*, *E. coli*, *Streptococcus viridans*, *Enterococcus spp*, *Pseudomonas*, and *Candida spp*. *Clostridium spp* particularly *clostridium septicum* play an important role and may be associated with increased mortality [17–19].

Clinical manifestations include right lower abdominal distention, abdominal cramps, nausea, vomiting, watery or bloody diarrhea sometimes with hematochezia, and fever. The symptoms usually develop after the 3rd week of chemotherapy [19].

The diagnosis is usually clinical based on the above symptoms. Computed tomography (CT) of the abdomen and pelvis can confirm the diagnosis and rule out complications such as pneumatosis intestinalis and perforation. CT may reveal colonic wall thickening and cecum dilation (Fig. 4). Plain abdominal x ray lacks sensitivity but may reveal dilation of the cecum and ascending colon with intramural gas [17, 19].

The treatment of typhlitis is initially conservative with bowel rest, nasogastric suction, and parenteral nutrition if necessary. Systemic antibiotics such as piperacillin tazobactam, or cefepime plus metronidazole or ceftazidime plus metronidazole, or meropenem, imipenem or doripenem are indicated. Surgical therapy is only indicated when clinical deterioration is imminent despite the above measures. Other indications for surgical therapy include persistent bleeding despite correction of coagulopathies or bowel perforation [19].

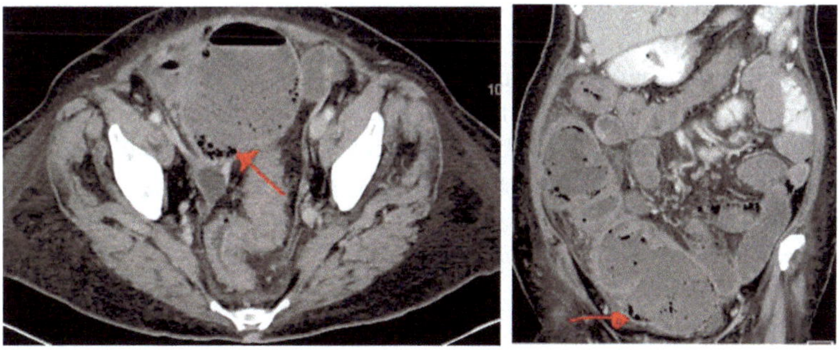

Fig. 4 CT of the abdomen and pelvis of a patient with neutropenic colitis with significantly dilated cecum and ascending colon. There is air within the bowel wall in the ascending colon to the level of the splenic flexure

Clostridium Difficile *Associated Disease*

Clostridium difficile associated disease is an important cause of morbidity and mortality in neutropenic patients. Chemotherapy, prophylactic antibiotics, mucositis, prolonged hospitalization, use of proton pump inhibitors, and immunosuppression predispose this population to develop *Clostridum difficile* associated disease. A multicenter survey reported that hospital acquired *Clostridium difficile* infection was twice as common in the cancer population compared with the general population [20].

The clinical diagnosis of *Clostridium difficile* associated disease represents a challenge in neutropenic patients because chemotherapy associated enteritis may have similar symptomatology. Some studies have shown that less than half of cancer patients with *C. diff* associated diarrhea have the classical symptoms including fever and abdominal pain [20].

The diagnosis of severe *Clostridium difficile* associated disease in neutropenic patients may be difficult to assess since these patients lack typical leukocytosis. In addition, they may have chronic kidney disease. In such patients, clinical judgment to treat as severe disease is a bedside decision.

Treatment and microbiologic diagnosis of *Clostridium difficile* in neutropenic patients follows the same recommendation as for non-neutropenic patients. Unfortunately, high risk neutropenic patients require prophylactic antibiotics which cannot be discontinued.

Either vancomycin or fidaxomicin is recommended over metronidazole for an initial episode of *Clostridium difficile*. If access to vancomycin or fidaxomicin is limited, then metronidazole for an initial episode of nonsevere *Clostridium difficile* infection is acceptable.

Oral vancomycin with or without intravenous metronidazole is the ideal treatment for severe and complicated *Clostridium difficile* associated disease. The use of probiotics to prevent Clostridium difficile associated disease is not endorsed by the Society for Healthcare Epidemiology of America (SHEA) and the Infectious Diseases Society of America (IDSA). In addition, there is concern for possible bloodstream infection with the use of probiotics in the neutropenic population [20, 21].

Classically, the length of treatment of *Clostridium difficile* associated disease is 10–14 days. However in neutropenic patients, treatment often needs to be continued while receiving prophylactic antibiotics to prevent relapse. In such cases, oral vancomycin 125 mg po bid can be used after 14 days of initial therapy while the patient remains on other antibiotics [22]. Metronidazole is not an ideal option for chronic prophylaxis to prevent *Clostridium difficile* because of the potential neurotoxicity when given beyond 28 days.

Fecal microbiota transplant is widely used in immunocompetent patients with recurrent *Clostridium difficile* associated diarrhea. In immunocompromised patients its use has not yet been accepted because of concern for donor related infections and bacterial translocation from the gastrointestinal tract to the blood stream [20].

Proctitis

Perirectal inflammation in neutropenic patients may occur as a result of mucosal inflammation from chemotherapy, diarrhea, bleeding hemorrhoids, or from perirectal furuncles. Perirectal wounds can later develop into rectal fissures or perirectal abscesses. Small peri-rectal wounds can lead to blood stream infections. Given the anatomic location, these infection are usually polymicrobial. Bacteria involved are often *E coli*, *Klebsiella spp*, *Pseudomonas spp*, *Enterobacter spp*, *Citrobacter spp*, *Proteus mirabilis*, *anaerobes spp*, *Enterococcus spp*, *Streptococcus viridans*, *Staphylococcus aureus* and *Candida spp*. Molds are rare but can also be found [16].

Symptoms include fever, severe peri-anal pain that can be associated with constipation.

Diagnosis is usually clinical. If there is any concern for peri-anal or peri-rectal abscess, a CT of the pelvis should be ordered to evaluate its extent. In such cases, surgical consultation is indicated. In neutropenic patients, the timing and indication of surgery may have to be balanced with the risks for bleeding and poor wound healing [23].

Systemic antibiotics such as vancomycin in addition to piperacillin tazobactam, cefepime with metronidazole, ceftazidime with metronidazole, meropenem, imipenem or doripenem are indicated. The initial antibiotic regimen can be narrowed to cover specific bacteria isolated once the patient is more stable and blood and perirectal cultures are finalized.

Diverticulitis

Diverticulitis results from microscopic or macroscopic perforation of a diverticulum due to local inflammation. In neutropenic patients with diverticulosis, the inflammation may be precipitated by enteritis from chemotherapy and constipation. Complicated diverticulitis can lead to abscess formation (Fig. 5), perforation and fecal peritonitis.

Given the above reasons, immunosuppressed patient are often at risk for complicated and recurrent diverticulitis.

The treatment of diverticulitis should include antibiotics to cover anaerobic organisms and enteric gram negative rods including Pseudomonas. Antibiotics such as piperacillin tazobactam, or cefepime plus metronidazole or ceftazidime plus metronidazole, or meropenem, imipenem or doripenem are indicated. A low threshold for surgical treatment in immunosuppressed patients is endorsed by the 2014 Guidelines by the American Society of Colon and Rectal Surgeons, but further study revealed increasing morbidity following surgical therapy in patients receiving chemotherapy [24, 25].

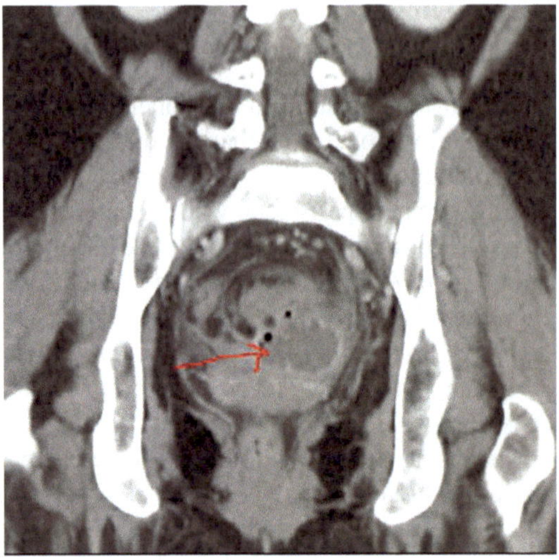

Fig. 5 CT of a patient with diverticulitis and sigmoid abscess

The decision of surgical treatment should be individualized balancing the risk vs benefits considering the acute illness, overall medical condition, chances of healing and or eradicating the infection with medical therapy alone.

Cholecystitis and Cholangitis

Cholangitis and cholecystitis in neutropenic patients just as in the general population results from cholelithiasis. It can also result from malignant lesions of the biliary tract. As a result, enteric gram negative rods, and anaerobic bacteria can translocate into the bloodstream causing sepsis.

The clinical symptoms include fever, right upper quadrant abdominal pain and jaundice if obstructive cholangitis is present. Treatment includes relieving the obstruction of the biliary tree if present and systemic antibiotics [26].

Antibiotics such as piperacillin tazobactam, or vancomycin and cefepime plus metronidazole or vancomycin and ceftazidime plus metronidazole, or vancomycin and meropenem, imipenem or doripenem are indicated.

Hepatitis

Hepatitis B virus (HBV) and hepatitis C (HCV) are very common viruses worldwide. In oncologic patients, HBV reactivation ranges between 30% and 80% depending the chemotherapy regimen.

The Center of Disease Control (CDC) recommends screening for HBV in all patients receiving cytotoxic or immunosuppressive therapy. Patients who have hepatitis B surface antigen (HBsAg) or who are hepatitis B core antibody (HBcAb) positive and receive chemotherapy regimens with anti CD20 agents, TNF alpha inhibitors, and anthracyclines are at higher risk for reactivation. In these patients HBV prophylaxis should be considered. Ideal regimens for HBV prophylaxis include tenofovir, entecavir adefovir and lamivudine [26–28].

HCV reactivation in cancer patients has not been well studied and little is known about the need for prophylaxis, but newer therapies can ensure cure in 12 weeks decreasing morbidity and mortality in this population. The National Comprehensive Cancer Network (NCCN) guidelines recommends that all patients receiving chemotherapy or immunosuppressive therapy should be screened and treated for HCV particularly if the life expectancy is greater than 12 months [26, 27].

Other viruses such as Cytomegalovirus (CMV), Herpes Simplex Virus (HSV), Varicella Zoster Virus (VZV) and Adenovirus can also cause severe hepatitis in neutropenic and immunosuppressed patients, but are rare outisde of the allogeneic stem cell transplant population . These infections are not within the scope of this chapter.

Genitourinary Tract Infections

Neutropenia, chemotherapy, mucosal inflammation and indwelling foley catheters increase the susceptibility for developing genitourinary infections (GU) infection. Although the pathogenesis is similar to the immunocompetent population, the infections are more frequent and severe in neutropenic patients.

Unfortunately, in this population, the diagnosis represents a challenge because the signs and symptoms of inflammation may be absent and the sensitivity of pyuria may be low [29].

The presence of a foley catheter increases the risk of bacteriuria 5–10% per day. The most common organisms that cause urinary tract infections include enteric gram negative rods such as *E coli, klebsiella pneumoniae*, and *Proteus mirabilis. Staphylococcus saprophyticus* is also a common pathogen [30].

In neutropenic patients, other bacteria such as *Enterococcus* and *Pseudomonas spp* can also cause GU infections. Rarely molds including *Fusarium spp* may be involved [31].

The treatment of urinary tract infections in neutropenic patients should be directed towards the isolated organism. The duration may be longer to prevent recurrent infection while the patient is still neutropenic.

Antimicrobial treatment should also be given for patients with prolonged and profound neutropenia and asymptomatic bacteriuria because of the high risk of bacteremia.

Hemorrhagic viral cystitis is an important cause of morbidity and mortality in transplant patients but is rarely seen in neutropenic patients without transplant. The viruses commonly involved are BK, Adenovirus, and CMV.

Key Points

Disease	Organisms	Antibiotics
Esophagitis	Candida, HSV, rarely CMV	Fluconazole if Candida. Famciclovir, or Valacyclovir. If HSV, and Ganciclovir if CMV.
Typhlitis, diverticulitis	*Klebsiella spp*, *E. coli*, *Streptococcus viridans*, *Enterococcus spp*, *Pseudomonas*, *Candida spp*, *Clostridium spp* and other anaerobes	Piperacillin tazobactam. Cefepime plus metronidazole. Ceftazidime plus Metronidazole. Meropenem, or Imipenem or Doripenem.
Proctitis	*E coli*, *Klebsiella spp*, *Pseudomonas spp*, *Enterobacter spp*, *Citrobacter spp*, *Proteus*, *anaerobes*, *Enterococcus spp*, *Streptococcus viridans*, *Staphylococcus aureus* and *Candida spp*. Molds are rare but can also be found	Vancomycin plus Piperacillin Tazobactam. Vancomycin plus Cefepime and Metronidazole. Vancomycin plus Ceftazidime and Metronidazole. Vancomycin and Meropenem, Imipenem or Doripenem until susceptibilities are available.
Clostridium difficile colitis	*Clostridium dificile*	Oral Vancomycin or Fidaxomicin. If access to Vancomycin or Fidaxomicin is limited, then Metronidazole for initial episode of nonsevere *Clostridium difficile* infection. Oral vancomycin with or without intravenous Metronidazole for severe and complicated *Clostridium difficile* associated disease.
Cholecystitis and Cholangitis	Enteric gram negative rods, anaerobic bacteria	Piperacillin tazobactam. Vancomycin and Cefepime plus Metronidazole. Vancomycin and Ceftazidime plus Metronidazole. Vancomycin and Meropenem, Imipenem or Doripenem

References

1. Komeno Y, Uryu H, Iwata Y, Hatada Y, Sakamoto J, Iihara K, et al. Esophageal candidiasis as the initial manifestation of acute myeloid leukemia. Int Med (Tokyo, Japan). 2015;54(23):3087–92.
2. Samonis G, Skordilis P, Maraki S, Datseris G, Toloudis P, Chatzinikolaou I, et al. Oropharyngeal candidiasis as a marker for esophageal candidiasis in patients with cancer. Clin Infect Dis. 1998;27(2):283–6.
3. Darouiche RO. Oropharyngeal and esophageal candidiasis in immunocompromised patients: treatment issues. Clin Infect Dis. 1998;26(2):259–72; quiz 73–4.
4. Pappas PG, Kauffman CA, Andes DR, Clancy CJ, Marr KA, Ostrosky-Zeichner L, et al. Executive summary: clinical practice guideline for the management of candidiasis: 2016 update by the Infectious Diseases Society of America. Clin Infect Dis. 2016;62(4):409–17.
5. Kadayakkara DK, Candelaria A, Kwak YE, Loeser C. Herpes simplex virus-2 esophagitis in a young immunocompetent adult. Case Rep Gastrointest Med. 2016;2016:7603484.
6. Canalejo Castrillero E, Garcia Duran F, Cabello N, Garcia Martinez J. Herpes esophagitis in healthy adults and adolescents: report of 3 cases and review of the literature. Medicine. 2010;89(4):204–10.
7. Harris J, Smith T, Preis J. Intractable hiccups due to herpetic esophagitis in an immunocompromised patient. IDCases. 2016;4:34–7.
8. Jazeron JF, Barbe C, Frobert E, Renois F, Talmud D, Brixi-Benmansour H, et al. Virological diagnosis of herpes simplex virus 1 esophagitis by quantitative real-time PCR assay. J Clin Microbiol. 2012;50(3):948–52.
9. Frobert E, Ooka T, Cortay JC, Lina B, Thouvenot D, Morfin F. Herpes simplex virus thymidine kinase mutations associated with resistance to acyclovir: a site-directed mutagenesis study. Antimicrob Agents Chemother. 2005;49(3):1055–9.
10. Wang HW, Kuo CJ, Lin WR, Hsu CM, Ho YP, Lin CJ, et al. The clinical characteristics and manifestations of cytomegalovirus esophagitis. Dis Esophagus. 2016;29(4):392–9.
11. Whitley RJ, Jacobson MA, Friedberg DN, Holland GN, Jabs DA, Dieterich DT, et al. Guidelines for the treatment of cytomegalovirus diseases in patients with AIDS in the era of potent antiretroviral therapy: recommendations of an international panel. International AIDS Society-USA. Arch Intern Med. 1998;158(9):957–69.
12. Goodgame RW. Gastrointestinal cytomegalovirus disease. Ann Intern Med. 1993;119(9):924–35.
13. Baroco AL, Oldfield EC. Gastrointestinal cytomegalovirus disease in the immunocompromised patient. Curr Gastroenterol Rep. 2008;10(4):409–16.
14. Bonatti H, Sifri CD, Larcher C, Schneeberger S, Kotton C, Geltner C. Use of cidofovir for cytomegalovirus disease refractory to ganciclovir in solid organ recipients. Surg Infect. 2017;18(2):128–36.
15. El Chaer F, Shah DP, Chemaly RF. How I treat resistant cytomegalovirus infection in hematopoietic cell transplantation recipients. Blood. 2016;128(23):2624–36.
16. Rolston KV, Bodey GP, Safdar A. Polymicrobial infection in patients with cancer: an underappreciated and underreported entity. Clin Infect Dis. 2007;45(2):228–33.
17. Rodrigues FG, Dasilva G, Wexner SD. Neutropenic enterocolitis. World J Gastroenterol. 2017;23(1):42–7.
18. Katz JA, Wagner ML, Gresik MV, Mahoney DH Jr, Fernbach DJ. Typhlitis. An 18-year experience and postmortem review. Cancer. 1990;65(4):1041–7.
19. Nesher L, Rolston KV. Neutropenic enterocolitis, a growing concern in the era of widespread use of aggressive chemotherapy. Clin Infect Dis. 2013;56(5):711–7.
20. Neemann K, Freifeld A. Clostridium difficile-associated diarrhea in the oncology patient. J Oncol Pract. 2017;13(1):25–30.
21. McDonald LC, Gerding DN, Johnson S, Bakken JS, Carroll KC, Coffin SE, et al. Clinical practice guidelines for clostridium difficile infection in adults and children: 2017 update by

the Infectious Diseases Society of America (IDSA) and Society for Healthcare Epidemiology of America (SHEA). Clin Infect Dis. 2018;6(7):987–94.
22. Van Hise NW, Bryant AM, Hennessey EK, Crannage AJ, Khoury JA, Manian FA. Efficacy of oral vancomycin in preventing recurrent clostridium difficile infection in patients treated with systemic antimicrobial agents. Clin Infect Dis. 2016;63(5):651–3.
23. Chen CY, Cheng A, Huang SY, Sheng WH, Liu JH, Ko BS, et al. Clinical and microbiological characteristics of perianal infections in adult patients with acute leukemia. PLoS One. 2013;8(4):e60624.
24. Feingold D, Steele SR, Lee S, Kaiser A, Boushey R, Buie WD, et al. Practice parameters for the treatment of sigmoid diverticulitis. Dis Colon Rectum. 2014;57(3):284–94.
25. Samdani T, Pieracci FM, Eachempati SR, Benarroch-Gampel J, Weiss A, Pietanza MC, et al. Colonic diverticulitis in chemotherapy patients: should operative indications change? A retrospective cohort study. Int J Surg. 2014;12(12):1489–94.
26. Rolston KV. Infections in cancer patients with solid tumors: a review. Infect Dis Ther. 2017;6(1):69–83.
27. Baden LR, Swaminathan S, Angarone M, Blouin G, Camins BC, Casper C, et al. Prevention and treatment of cancer-related infections, version 2.2016, NCCN clinical practice guidelines in oncology. J Natl Compr Canc Netw. 2016;14(7):882–913.
28. Mindikoglu AL, Regev A, Schiff ER. Hepatitis B virus reactivation after cytotoxic chemotherapy: the disease and its prevention. Clin Gastroenterol Hepatol. 2006;4(9):1076–81.
29. Klaassen IL, de Haas V, van Wijk JA, Kaspers GJ, Bijlsma M, Bokenkamp A. Pyuria is absent during urinary tract infections in neutropenic patients. Pediatr Blood Cancer. 2011;56(5):868–70.
30. Gupta K, Hooton TM, Naber KG, Wullt B, Colgan R, Miller LG, et al. International clinical practice guidelines for the treatment of acute uncomplicated cystitis and pyelonephritis in women: a 2010 update by the Infectious Diseases Society of America and the European Society for Microbiology and Infectious Diseases. Clin Infect Dis. 2011;52(5):e103–20.
31. Su H, Zhang Q, Li L, Zhao Y, Zhu J, Zhu M. Urinary tract infection (UTI) caused by fusarium proliferatum in an agranulocytosis patient and a review of published reports. Mycopathologia. 2016;181(1–2):131–5.

Skin Infections

Nancy Rihana and Mindy Sampson

Abstract Cutaneous infections are common in immunocompromised patients. Neutropenia predisposes patients to fungal, bacterial and viral infections. Antibacterial antifungal and antiviral prophylaxis have caused a significant reduction in some of these infections.

There are two main types of cutaneous infections: primary cutaneous infections and cutaneous manifestations of a disseminated infection. In the latter, skin lesions may be the window to disseminated bloodstream infection and the first and only evidence of a disseminated life threatening infection.

The diagnosis may be at your fingertips; therefore a thorough skin exam is the clue. However, it's also important to know the characteristic lesions associated with different infections. It will help expedite diagnosis so appropriate treatment is initiated promptly in neutropenic patients, which can be lifesaving.

In a retrospective study of 43 neutropenic febrile patients with cutaneous lesions, fungal infections were the most frequent, and nodular lesions on the lower extremities were the most prevalent (Naorungroj and Aiempanakit, J Am Acad Dermatol 74:AB166, 2016).

Skin biopsy for pathological study and culture remains the gold standard and should be obtained early to confirm the suspected diagnosis. In these immunocompromised patients the inflammatory response is altered by either the primary disease or its treatment. Therefore, routine pathogens may present in an atypical fashion, with diminished or absent induration, erythema, or pustulation in response to bacterial resulting cutaneous infection without typical cellulitis (Urabe, Clin Infect Dis 39:S53–S55, 2004). Skin lesions are evaluated not only by morphology, but also in the context of the clinical setting and biopsy result. The skin biopsy is inexpensive, relatively noninvasive and without contraindication, and may avoid the need for more invasive procedures such an open lung biopsy (Grossman, et al., Cutaneous manifestations of infection in the immunocompromised host. Springer Science+Business Media, LLC, New York, 2012).

N. Rihana (✉) · M. Sampson
University of South Florida, Tampa, FL, USA
e-mail: nrihana@health.usf.edu

A. P. Velez et al. (eds.), *Infections in Neutropenic Cancer Patients*,
https://doi.org/10.1007/978-3-030-21859-1_5

In addition to antimicrobial therapy, surgery should not be postponed in the face of progressive skin and soft tissue infection in this population (Brzozowski and Ross, J Hand Surg Br 22:679–680, 1997).

Keywords Ecthyma gangrenosum · Bullous cellulitis · Fulminant necrotizing infections · Spontaneous clostridial myonecrosis · Purplish discoloration · Crepitation · Necrotizing enterocolitis · Subcutaneous nodules · Disseminated cutaneous mycobacterium · knife-cut sign · Herpetic whitlow · Disseminated HZ

Bacterial Infections

Gram Negative Bacteria

Neutropenia is one of the major risk factors for gram-negative cellulitis. We will review the main gram negative pathogens and their cutaneous manifestations in this population.

Pseudomonas aeruginosa, usually a nosocomial pathogen has emerged as a common cause of infection in immunocompromised patients; most often in neutropenic leukemics during chemotherapy. The routine use of anti-pseudomona antimicrobial prophylaxis in cancer patients with prolonged neutropenia has reduced the overall incidence of pseudomonal infections. However the emergence fluroquinolone resistant gram negatives including Pseudomonas remains an important threat in neutropenic patients. Pseudomonas can invade through areas of micro erosions especially over intravenous, urinary catheters, decubital ulcerations and thermic damage [1].

Cutaneous lesions occur in 30% of cases of Pseudomonas bacteremia [2]. The site of origin of the Pseudomonas is most commonly the respiratory or genitourinary tract. P. aeruginosa infection can also be acquired from a humid environment including showers, sinks, and flower vases.

The dermatologic manifestations of Pseudomonas sepsis include ecthyma gangrenosum, hemorrhagic bullae, necrotizing/gangrenous or bullous cellulitis, painful vesicular lesions, and small papules on the trunk resembling rose spots of typhoid fever, grouped petechiae, erysipelas-like lesions with hyperesthesia, erythematous or violaceous subcutaneous painful nodules, and necrotizing or malignant external otitis [3].

Ecthyma gangrenosum (EG) has classically been considered a pathognomonic sign of Pseudomonas aeruginosa septicemia, although it can be reported with multiple other gram-negative bacterial, fungal, and viral infections in the immunocompromised host. It can occur as single or multiple lesions. Most cases of ecthyma gangrenosum have been associated with septicemia, but it can also occur in the absence of Pseudomonas bacteremia. The most common sites for ecthyma gangrenosum are the gluteal, perineal area, axillary and extremities [4].

It begins as an area of erythema and edema that progresses to hemorrhagic bullae that rupture, evolving into a painless central blackish gray necrotic area (eschar) surrounded by an erythematous halo. It grows up to several centimeters in diameter over 12–24 h. The necrosis may extend as deep as muscle. Pus is minimal. Lesions at various stages of development may be present at different sites in the same patient [3]. Ulcerations are sensitive on palpation [1]. It is assumed that necrosis of the skin is caused by *Pseudomonas* elastase which destroys elastic lamina of the blood vessels and allows liberation of the pathogen into the subcutaneous tissues [5] (Fig. 1).

The pathologic hallmark of EC is vasculitis sparing the intima and without thrombosis which distinguishes it from other forms of bacterial vasculitis in which septic intraluminal thrombi attach to bacteria and invade the endothelium [4].

E. Coli, is a common cause of cellulitis in the immunocompromised host that is impossible to distinguish from streptococcal cellulitis. It is rapidly progressive and limb threatening if appropriate antibiotic are not started promptly [3, 6]. E. coli may also produce abscesses anywhere in the body but mainly cause perirectal phlegmon in neutropenic patients.

Ecthyma gangrenosum described above, is considered pathognomonic for Pseudomonas aeruginosa but has also been described with multiple other gram-negative organisms including E. coli, E. cloacae, Klebsiella, Serratia, Citrobacter, Morganella, and Stenotrophomonas [3, 7–11]

Aeromonas species are gram-negative, non-sporulating facultative anaerobic bacillus found in brackish or fresh water lakes, streams and soils. They have also been recovered from chlorinated tap water, including hospital water supplies. It may be isolated as well from stools of asymptomatic carriers. Among patients with cancer, Aeromonas septicemia is more likely to occur in leukemic patients and its associated with water related activities in only 10% cases but is nosocomially acquired in 60% [12]. About 20–30% of infections are associated with skin lesions.

In immunosuppressed patients, Aeromonas can cause various infections that are likely to be fatal including severe cellulitis, fulminant necrotizing infections, and ecthyma gangrenosum. Myonecrosis and gas production have occurred with Aeromonas and can simulate clostridial gas gangrene [3].

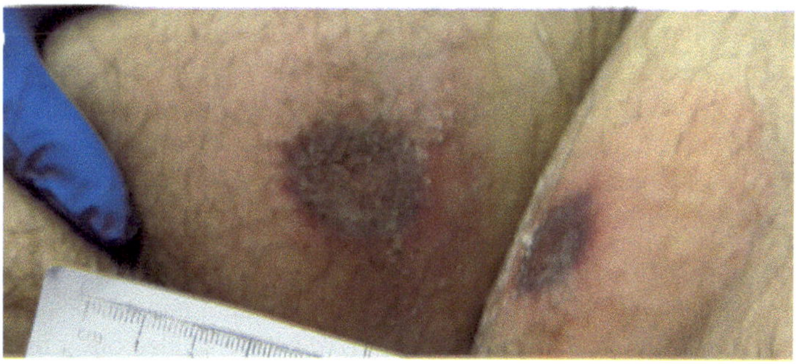

Fig. 1 Ecthyma gangrenosum secondary to Pseudomonas aeruginosa in a neutropenic patient after induction therapy for acute myelogeneous leukemia

Aeromonas infections of freshwater traumatic wounds after water related activities such as fishing or swimming cause a rapidly progressive cellulitis that develops within 8–48 h after trauma followed by suppuration and necrosis around the wound, myonecrosis and sometimes osteomyelitis. It often requires surgical debridement in addition to antibiotic therapy [4].

Chromobacterium violaceum is a rare but frequently fatal infection. Its an anaerobic gram-negative rod that is commonly found in soil and water in tropical and sub-tropical climates between latitudes 35° north and 35° south. Cutaneous infection is rare and usually occurs with exposure of broken or injured skin to contaminated muddy or stagnant water or soil in patients with neutrophil dysfunction or HIV infection. Infection in the skin tends to present with cellulitis, pustules, ulcers, or abscesses accompanied by severe systemic symptoms [3].

Gram Positive Bacteria

Over the course of the last several decades, the frequency with which gram-positive bacteria have been isolated from neutropenic patients with cancer has increased [13]. We will review the main gram positive pathogens that lead to cutaneous involvement in neutropenic patients.

Bacillus cereus commonly presents in a neutropenic patient as a single painful vesicle, pustule, or bulla on a digit or extremities with rapidly spreading cellulitis during the spring and summer. The bulla may become necrotic and develop a black eschar. It's usually associated with systemic toxicity [3]. Gram stain of the aspirate smear demostrates large Gram-positive rods, which may be mistaken for Clostridium infection and treated with penicillin. B. cereus and B subtilus cause most of the infections. About half of these infections arise at sites of indwelling intravascular catheters [4]. occasionally widely disseminated blood stream infections may occur including endocarditis and brain abscess [14–16].

Clostridium species account for 30% of anaerobic bacteremias in all cancer patients [17]. It tends to cause a fulminant infection in neutropenic patients. Sixty percent of the isolated cases are secondary to Clostridium perfringens and 30% by Clostridium septicum. Clostridium perfringens is usually part of the colonic flora while C. septicum is typically found in soil and animals, but is not normal human flora [3]. Forty percent of the clostridium infections are polymicrobial, which indicates the gastrointestinal tract as the source of these infections [17].

Two types of cutaneous manifestation have been described in neutropenic patients: spontaneous, non-traumatic gas gangrene, and spreading cellulitis [4].

(a) Spontaneous clostridial myonecrosis (gas gangrene) most commonly associated with a silent colon carcinoma, an underlying hematologic tumor or neutrophil dysfunction [3]. Its is clinically characterized by the sudden onset of excruciating pain in the involved site- usually the leg esp. if associated with abdominal involvement. The swelling is rapidly progressive, associated with purplish/bronze discoloration and blister formation- usually hemorrhagic. Involvement of underlying muscle is always more extensive than the evident skin involvement. The blister serosanguinous fluid will contain GPR, but inflammatory cells are infrequent [4]. Pathology: there is cell lysis and gas formation in connective tissue and muscle with minimal inflammation [4].

The diagnosis of clostridial myonecrosis requires a high index of suspicion, since the infection spreads rapidly and death may occur within 24–48 h. Gram stain of a bulla allows for a timely diagnosis. Anaerobic cultures should be sent to determine appropriate antibiotic use. Imaging with X-ray or computed tomography (CT) scan can demonstrate soft tissue gas (a late finding) and help determine the extent of infection [3].

(b) Spreading cellulitis with clostridial septicemia is a fulminant infection in neutropenic patients. A small area of purplish discoloration develops, often on the flank or abdominal wall. The lesion will expand rapidly over several hours, and more lesions appear in other areas. As it progresses, the lesions turn into brownish to blackish color with blister formation and crepitation. Clostridium can be captured in the fluid, but without inflammatory cells [4].

Clostridium septicum has been associated with necrotizing enterocolitis (typhlitis), which typically is a fulminant infection of the intestines in neutropenic patients [18].

Corynebacterium jeikeium (C. jeikeium) Corynebacterium species are part of the normal skin flora. The most common sites of colonization by C. jeikeium are the perineum, rectal, inguinal and axillary areas. Corynebacteria species rarely cause infection. Infections due to C. jeikeium are mainly seen in immunosuppressed patients, especially those with neutropenia and indwelling catheters [19].

Primary cutaneous infection with C. jeikeium occurs at breaks in the skin barrier due to bone marrow biopsy, intravascular catheter insertion, groin or perirectal areas (anal fissures) which serve as a portal of entry into the bloodstream, leading to septicemia. Primary skin lesions typically present as cellulitis or wound infection [20].

Secondary skin and soft tissue infections with C. jeikeium develop in almost 30–50% of neutropenic patient with C jeikeium bacteremia [4]. It may present as single to multiple, nontender, noninflamed 2 × 2 cm subcutaneous nodules that do not spontaneously drain but are purulent upon surgical drainage [19]; bright red, non-blanching papules with satellite petechiae and central necrosis or pustulation on the trunk and/or extremities [20].

Staphylococci species are frequent colonizers of normal skin but commonly infect immunocompromised individuals. Leukopenic patients are at greatest risk for infection. Common infections include impetigo, furuncles, carbuncles, ecthyma, folliculitis, cellulitis etc. In immunocompromised patient, vesicle or bullous eruption can be seen [3].

Streptococcal infections in bone marrow transplant (BMT) recipients and acute leukemia patients are serious and may be clinically atypical [4]. Group A or Group B streptococcus cutaneous manifestations include erysipelas/cellulitis in only 25%, the rest of the cases are infections of wounds or ulcers, myositis, necrotizing fasciitis, and toxic shock syndrome.

Viridans group streptococci (VGS) are part of the normal microbial flora of humans, risk factors for invasive disease is mucositis and neutropenia.

A case control study of VGS sepsis was done at the University of Texas M. D. Anderson Cancer Center in Houston, where controls were randomly selected from patients with other Gram-positive septicemia. Flushing of the face and a rash occurred in nearly 60% of these patients but were uncommon in the control group. The rash was usually erythematous maculopapular, beginning on the trunk and progressing to the face and extremities compatible with toxic shock syndrome picture. In 25% of the cases, the rash resulted in desquamation of the palms and soles 1–2 weeks later. Ten percent of the patients developed ARDS, shock, or renal failure and died despite more than 4 days of vancomycin therapy. The patients with VSG had a higher rate of oral mucositis, BMT, and severe neutropenia <100, on antacid or H2 antagonist therapy, and parenteral nutrition [4, 21].

Mycobacteria

Mycobacterial cutaneous infection occurs as a result of direct inoculation from an exogenous source, or through contiguous or hematogenous spread. Cutaneous mycobacteria can exhibit a large spectrum of morphological presentation. Infection may be caused by Mycobacterium tuberculosis (MTb), Mycobacterium avium intracellulare complex (MAC), and other non-tuberculous mycobacteria (NTM) including rapidly growing mycobacteria (RGM), although MTb is commonly seen in HIV patients those undergoing solid organ transplant.

Tuberculosis in neutropenic patients is one of the most serious opportunistic infections encountered. Cutaneous miliary tuberculosis presents as erythematous to brown papules, which can become vesicular or pustular. The tiny vesicles or pustules rupture and form a central crust on the papule. Removal of the crust leaves a minute but sharply defined umbilication [3].

Pathology results are characterized by the absence of a granulomatous response, giant cells, and true caseating granulomas [6]. An acid-fast stain (if the diagnosis is considered and the stain requested) usually shows numerous acid-fast bacilli (AFB) seen quite easily [3].

NTM are ubiquitous in the environment and reside in soil and water. Of the over 150 NTM species, only ~25 are known to cause disease in humans [22]. Skin and soft tissue infections are most commonly caused by *Mycobacterium marinum* and *Mycobacterium ulcerans*, which are both slowly growing mycobacteria [23].

In the immunocompromised, the typical history of previous trauma or surgery is absent, thus cutaneous *Mycobacteria* infection are most probably the result of hematogenic dissemination, resulting in multiple skin lesions. This clinical entity is well described in patients with T cell mediated immunodeficiency such as AIDS, solid organ and bone marrow transplant patients, but infrequently in patients with hematological malignancies, either with or without neutropenia [24].

Case studies described highlight the variety of immune system dysfunction (T-cell, humoral, or granulocyte-related) which combined may have predisposed to the disseminated NTM in neutropenic patients [13, 25]. Chronic indwelling central venous catheter-related infection is one of the most common risk factor for disseminated nontuberculous mycobacterial infection [26].

The lesions are usually more extensive in the immunosuppressed population, nonspecific and heterogeneous. They range from panniculitis (Fig. 2), single to widespread nodules, sinus tracts, nonhealing ulcers, subcutaneous abscesses, or erythematous plaques (Fig. 3) [3].

Mycobacterium malmoense, a slow-growing mycobacteria may cause cutaneous lesions that were described in a 75 year old neutropenic man with myelodysplastic syndrome, who was also receiving corticosteroids. He developed papulokeratotic pinkish nodules lesions in a sporotrichoid distribution on the arm that later ulcerated and some became necrotic [27].

Mycobacterium avium-intracellulare complex (MAC), is a common opportunistic pathogen in AIDS patients and patients with cell medicated immunodeficiency mainly, it can also cause infections in neutropenic patients. The clinical manifestations include widespread erythematous tender nodules on the upper, and lower extremities, chest and abdomen that can ulcerate (Fig. 2). The infection is usually associated with bacteremia and cavitary lung lesions may also be present. Skin biopsy demonstrates areas of dermal and subcutaneous necrosis with numerous acid-fast bacilli [3].

Mycobacterium fortuitum, Mycobacterium abscessus, and Mycobacterium chelonae are collectively referred to as rapidly growing mycobacteria (RGM). These environmental pathogens may cause skin infections that usually occur following trauma or surgical procedures and injections, which is usually not present in immunocompromised patients. M. fortuitum infection is more common in immunocompetent patients, while M. chelonae and M abscessus more often infects immunocompromised patients [3].

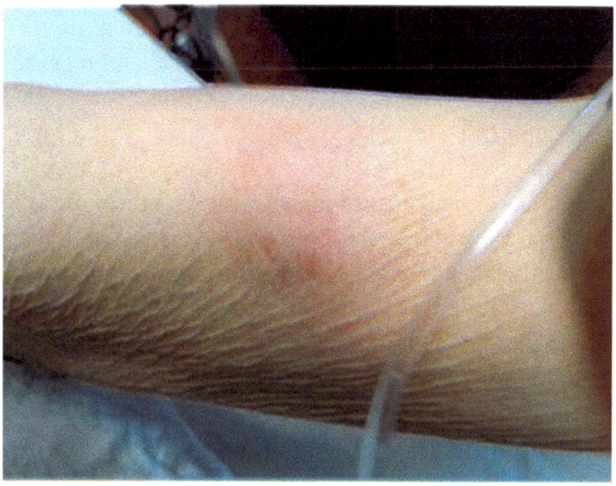

Fig. 2 Indurated tender red lesions on the extremities of an immunocompromised patient – skin biopsy was consistent with infectious panniculitis secondary to Mycobacterium chelonae

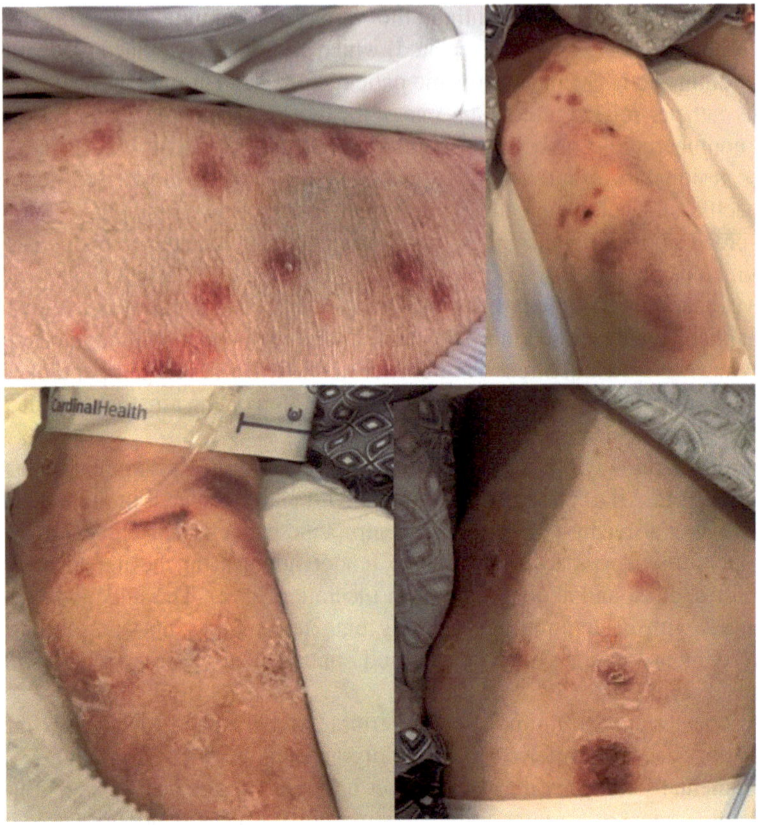

Fig. 3 Disseminated mycobacterium avium intracellulare complex in neutropenic patients

Disseminated cutaneous *Mycobacterium chelonae* infection in neutropenic patients can cause neutropenic fever and multiple dusky red to purple, tender, subcutaneous nodules on the face, arms, and legs, resulting in firm purple ulcerating nodules. Within weeks, the nodules can developed larger plaques that can ulcerate [25].

It is essential to maintain a high index of suspicion for atypical mycobacterial infection, as acid-fast organisms may be difficult to identify on histologic sections, and many of these fastidious pathogens are challenging to grow in culture, often requiring weeks for the culture to turn positive, and in some cases requiring specific media. Polymerase chain reaction (PCR) is an emerging technique, which may aid in the diagnosis of mycobacterial infections. Speciation of the offending organism is crucial, as the antibiotic susceptibility profiles differ among the organisms and are essential to achieving therapeutic success [3].

Viral Infections

Neutrophils are not the primary defense against viral infections. However hematologic malignancy is the most prevalent background of neutropenic patients with cutaneous lesions 95.3% based on a retrospective review from 2009–2014 [28]. In this population, the combination of dysfuction of different parts of the immune system provides sufficient opportunity for viruses such as *herpesiviridae* to reactivate and cause disseminated infection [13].

Herpes Simplex Virus

Infections caused by herpes simplex virus (HSV) are exceedingly common in-patient with acute leukemia and post bone marrow transplant [4].

They are divided into primary and secondary (recurrent) forms, which are self-limited in normal hosts. In the majority of immunocompromised hosts, the HSV infection is not primary but rather reactivation of latent HSV.

Most herpetic infections involve the oral mucosa, lips, and nares. Genital lesions are less common [4]. Any periorificial ulceration in the immunocompromised host should be considered herpes simplex until proven otherwise.

Symptoms such as paresthesia, burning sensation or pruritus precede the lesions. They begin as vesicles that rupture spontaneously, leaving ulcerations that enlarge, coalesce and become encrusted. Infection often follows a chronic course in immunosuppressed patients, resulting in larger, deeper, painful necrotic erosive lesions known as phagedena. Superinfection by bacteria or fungi, esp. by Staphylococcus aureus may occur, which may distort the initial appearance, resulting in misdiagnosis. Healing typically occurs within 1 week in normal hosts, but may take up to 5 weeks in immunocompromised patients [3, 4].

Intraoral HSV can present as ulcerations with polycyclic borders, linear fissures on the tongue known as herpetic geometric glossitis. The break of mucosal integrity provides a portal of invasion by both pathogenic and normal microbial flora inhabiting the mouth. Other variant of atypical herpes simplex virus infection is deep linear fissures in the skin folds (inframammary, infra-abdominal, inguinal, or vulvar) termed the "knife-cut sign", and bilateral mutidigit herpetic whitlow (Fig. 4) reported in a patient after receiving chemotherapy for chronic lymphocytic leukemia (CLL) [3].

Both oral and intravenous acyclovir has been effective in preventing HSV infection in patients with acute leukemia and BMT recipients.

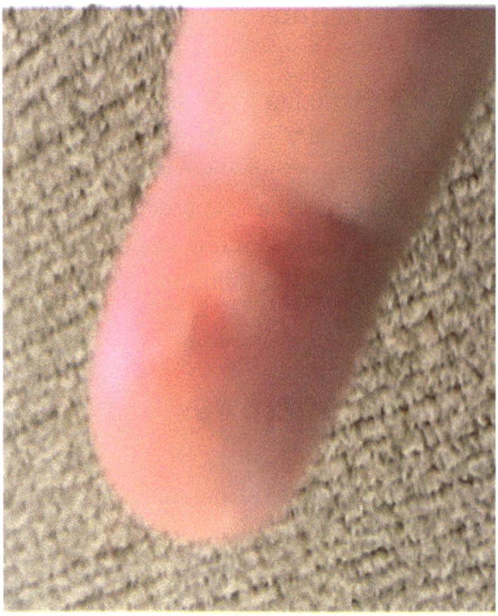

Fig. 4 Herpetic whitlow

Herpes Zoster Virus

Herpes zoster (HZ) represents reactivation of the varicella-zoster (VZ) virus. Following the primary varicella infection (chicken pox), the virus remains dormant in a dorsal root ganglion or a cranial nerve ganglion. Reactivation occurs as herpes zoster with cutaneous vesicles and dermatomal pain. The skin lesions of VZ in the immunocompromised host occur in three forms: (a) dermatomal HZ (which may be less than 3 contiguous dermatomes), (b) disseminated HZ and (c) chronic HZ or recurrent HZ. In patients with malignant disease, the incidence of HZ is further increased: highest in lymphoreticular disorders, Hodgkin's disease, then non-Hodgkin's lymphomas, followed by solid tumors, particularly small cell carcinoma of the lung [29] (Fig. 5).

Cytomegalovirus (CMV)

CMV (HHV-5) is a common human viral infection affecting 40–100% of adults worldwide. Acute infections are often asymptomatic, but once the infection is acquired, there is a lifelong latency along with the risk of intermittent reactivation. CMV disease is due to reactivation of latent virus following iatrogenic immunosuppression in organ transplantation, and cancer chemotherapy. Skin manifestations of CMV are rare in any setting, and very nonspecific (exanthematous, maculopapular, or morbilliform eruptions) and therefore diagnosis is often delayed. The cardinal manifestation of CMV infection in the skin is a chronic painful ulcer of the anal, perianal, or anogenital area. Although uncommon, oral manifestations of CMV

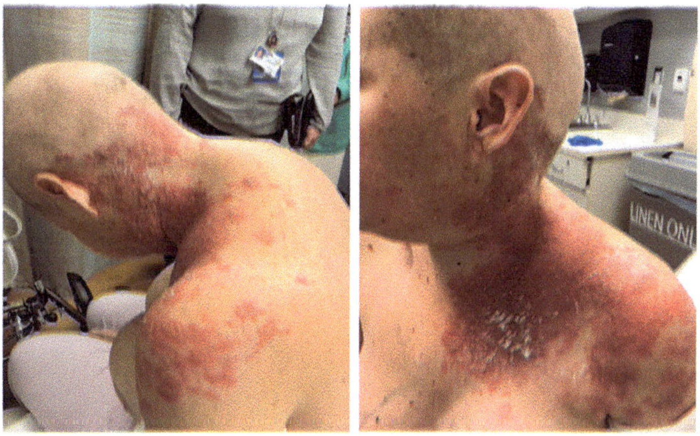

Fig. 5 Disseminated zoster in a neutropenic patient with acute myelogeneous leukemia

infection have included painful erosions or ulcers of the tongue, buccal mucosa, and pharynx. Skin biopsy will confirm the diagnosis by demonstrating the characteristic large intranuclear inclusions with a surrounding halo, or "owl's eye" characteristic of CMV. The diagnosis is confirmed with immunoperoxidase stain [3].

Fungal Infections

There are many fungi including yeast and mold, which are of medical importance, particularly in the immunocompromised population. Patients with hematologic malignancies and those receiving chemotherapy are at highest risk [30]. Fungal infections have many clinical presentations including dermatologic manifestations. These infections can be localized after local trauma, progress to invasive disease or dissemination, or result from hematogenous infection.

Candida

Superficial cutaneous *Candida* infections such as intertrigo and vaginitis present similarly to immunocompetent patients [30]. However, they may be more common in patients who require systemic antibiotics or steroids during their oncologic treatment. Most superficial infections can be treated with topical anti-fungal [31].

Disseminated candidiasis can occur in neutropenic and non-neutropenic populations. The portal of entry is typically via gastrointestinal translocation or introduction from a central line. In patients with hematologic malignancies and stem-cell transplantation, non-*albicans* species predominate including *C. glabrata*, *C. krusei* and *C. tropicalis* [32–36]. In solid tumors, approximately half of disseminated can-

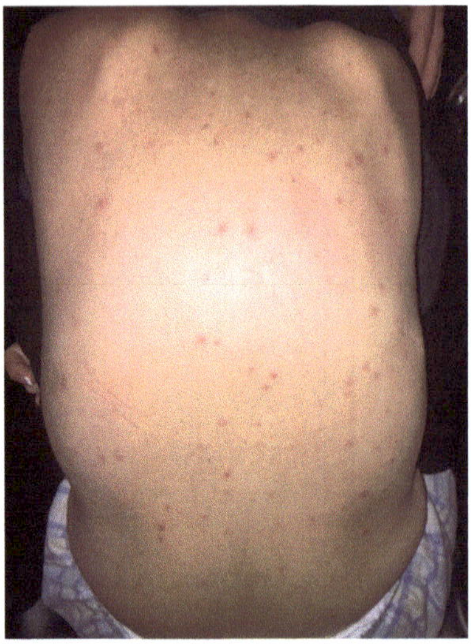

Fig. 6 Scattered papules of the back in a patient with disseminated *Candida tropicalis* in the setting of acute myelogenous leukemia and neutropenia

didiasis is secondary to *C. albicans* [32]. The epidemiology of these infections is likely related to the choice of fungal prophylaxis and resistance patterns of non-*albicans* species [34]. The frequency of cutaneous manifestations in the setting of candidemia is reported to occur in 11–44% of cases [34]. The typical skin lesions are 5–10 mm pink papules, which rarely lead to eschar formation or skin necrosis. There are often numerous papules involving the trunk and proximal extremities [30]. Some lesions may be purpuric, especially if thrombocytopenia is also present [34]. Mortality associated with candidemia has been reported to be over 50%, therefore prompt recognition of skin lesions and initiation of empiric treatment is important [35]. Diagnostics can be challenging, positive blood cultures occur in less than 50% of the cases. It is important to consider obtaining tissue for histopathology and culture or using novel non-culture diagnostics. Histology typically shows fungal elements including pseudohyphae, hyphae and yeast within the dermis or blood vessels [34]. An echinocandin such as micafungin is recommended as empiric treatment in most patients [31] (Fig. 6).

Fusarium

Skin manifestations occur in up to 70% of patients with Fusariosis and can present as a localized or disseminated infection [36]. Neutropenic patients with hematologic malignancies are at high risk for these mold infections [37]. An important clinical presentation of localized fusarium infection in the neutropenic population is fungal paronychia, which presents as erythema and swelling of the periungal skin [30]. Fungal paronychia should be suspected in neutropenic patients who have underlying onychomycosis, develop an eschar, and do not improve on systemic antibiotics [30]. Infection may be preceded by minor trauma [38]. Local infections can lead to fungemia and disseminated infection. Disseminated *Fusarium* infection typically presents as multiple erythematous papules or nodules, which can develop central necrosis or targetoid appearance. They often present at different stages of evolution and are widely distributed on the trunk and extremities [36].

Skin biopsy with histopathology and culture are helpful in securing a diagnosis. Histology will show ballooning branching septated hyphae, which can invade capillaries and blood vessels [39]. Skin lesions may appear before systemic symptoms develop or blood cultures become positive [30]. Unlike other disseminated mold infections, blood cultures are often positive in disseminated Fusariosis and should be collected when Fusarium is suspected [37]. Empiric treatment with liposomal amphotericin B is recommended [40]. More details about therapy please refer to the chapter titled fungal infections (Figs. 7, 8, and 9).

Aspergillus

Although aspergillus is one of the most common etiologies of invasive fungal infections in patients with underlying malignancies, dermatologic manifestations occurs in less than 5% of cases [41, 42]. Cutaneous involvement can present as a localized infection by direct skin inoculation or via hematogenous dissemination. Blood cultures are typically negative in disseminated infection therefore it is recommended to obtain tissue biopsy with culture and histopathology. Skin manifestations are similar to Fusarium infections. Primary or localized lesions can present as cellulitis with focal erythema and swelling that can progress leading to the formation of bullae, necrotic ulcers and eschars. Invasive fungal sinusitis secondary to *Aspergillus* sp. can also extend to the skin leading to facial cellulitis; this is covered in further detail in the chapter about fungal infections. Disseminated infection typically presents as scattered erythematous papules or nodules [30, 41]. Histology will show septated narrow hyphae with 45° branching and club-shaped pseudohyphae [43]. Treatment with

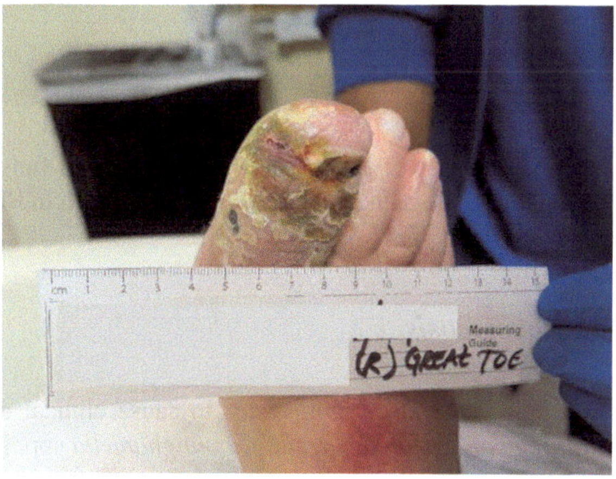

Fig. 7 Paronychia and cellulitis secondary to *Fusarium sp.* in a patient with acute myelogenous leukemia and prolonged neutropenia

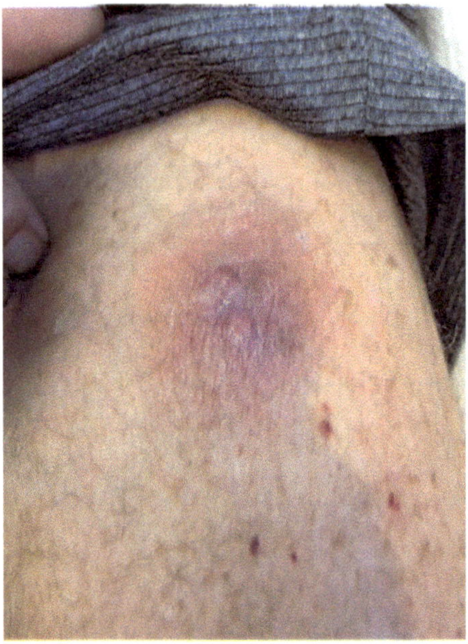

Fig. 8 Erythematous nodules with surrounding erythema in a patient with acute myelogenous leukemia and disseminated *Fusarium*

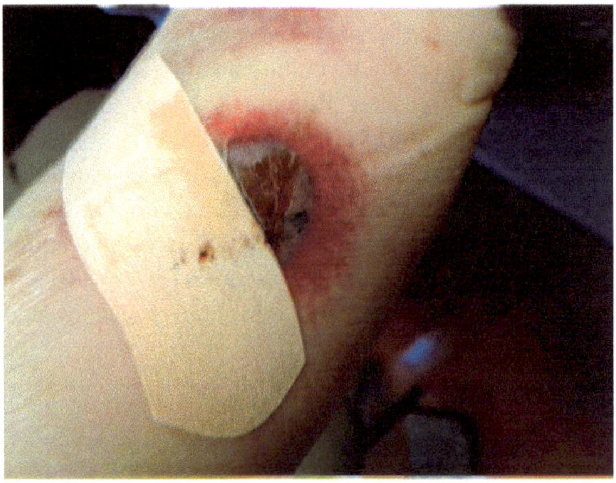

Fig. 9 Necrotic eschar with surrounding petechial erythema secondary to localized *Fusarium* infection in a patient with underlying B-cell lymphoma

triazoles such as voriconazole is the preferred anti-fungal unless there is a contraindication to this class and then liposomal amphotericin B would be recommended [44].

Mucormycosis

The most common Zygomycetes to cause clinical disease are *Rhizopus*, *Mucor*, *Rhizomucor*, *Lichtheimia,* and *Cunninghamella* spp. [45]. In patients with underlying malignancy, the primary site of mucormycosis is cutaneous in 12% of cases

[46]. Unlike other fungal infections, cutaneous mucormycosis most often occurs by direct inoculation rather than dissemination. Skin lesions may begin as a small erythematous macule but typically develop a black necrotic eschar with surrounding erythema and swelling. If there is concern for disseminated disease it is important to look for metastatic skin lesions [47]. Patients with rhinocerebral mucormycosis may present with orbital or facial cellulitis with a classic black necrotic eschar [45]. Obtaining tissue histopathology with culture is essential for diagnosis. Histologic examination will show broad non septate hyphae branching at 90° [43]. There may be vascular invasion leading to thrombosis and infarction [47]. Liposomal amphotericin B is treatment of choice [48].

Other Fungi

There are several other fungal infections that are less common but also important to consider in the evaluation of a cancer patient with a rash. Geographic location and previous travel can increase risk for endemic fungal infections.

Histoplasmosis is endemic in the Ohio River valley and parts of Central America. Cutaneous lesions typically present in cases of disseminated disease and often mimic other dermatologic infections due its' ability to manifest with many skin findings including papules, plaques, nodules, ulcers or pustules. Histopathology typically shows granulomas with lymphohistiocytic infiltrates and yeast within or outside macrophages [49].

Blastomycosis can be found in the Ohio and Mississippi river valleys and in the southeastern United States [50]. Skin lesions begin as an erythematous papule and evolve into a scaling or vegetative plaque. Histopathology may show pseudoepitheliomatous hyperplasia with neutrophilic abscesses or noncaseating granulomas. Tissue culture will reveal a thick-walled yeast with broad-based budding [51, 52].

Coccidiomycosis is found in the southwestern United States and can present with cutaneous findings when dissemination or reactivation occurs. Like histoplasmosis, disseminated coccidomycosis can present in many cutaneous forms including papules, plaques, nodules and ulcers. Histopathologic examination can show granulomatous or suppurative inflammation with numerous eosinophils. Coccidiomycosis can also result in reactive skin eruptions such as erythema nodosum, sweet's syndrome, interstitial granulomatous dermatitis, and exanthems. These presentations typically occur in the setting of pulmonary coccidiomycosis. Histopathology for reactive eruptions is variable depending on the skin manifestation and will have sterile tissue culture [53].

Cryptococcus spp. are encapsulated yeast, which are ubiquitous in the environment, often being found in the soil and pigeon droppings. These infections are commonly reported in the HIV population however they can occur in other immunocompromising conditions including malignancies. Like many other cutaneous fungal infections, skin lesions are polymorphous. Cutaneous findings can represent primary infection but most often occur in the setting of disseminated disease.

Therefore it is important to look for other organ involvement when cutaneous cryptococcal infection is diagnosed [54]. Obtaining histopathology with tissue culture is essential for diagnosis, using stains such as mucicarmine and alcian blue to identify the capsule [55].

Non Infectious Differential

Although it is always important to consider infectious dermatologic etiologies in cancer patients who present with a rash, there are also several non-infectious skin diseases that are important to recognize. Cancers themselves can cause unique skin pathology however there are also paraneoplastic and inflammatory skin disorders that can occur secondary to malignancies. Obtaining a thorough history and review of medications can assist with determining the diagnosis but skin biopsy is usually necessary given many diseases have similar findings on clinical examination.

Leukemia cutis

Leukemia cutis (LC) is an extra-medullary presentation of leukemia which is due to the invasion of malignant cells into the skin [56]. LC is most commonly associated with AML but can also occur with other underlying myeloid disorders and rarely presents without bone marrow involvement. Typical skin findings are erythematous or violaceous papules, nodules or plaques. The lesions have also been described as rubbery or shiny and may present with bullae [57, 58]. They can be pruritic but are usually not painful. Skin biopsy with immunohistochemical analysis is essential for diagnosis [59]. Histopathology will show leukemic cells, typically myeloblasts, invading the dermis. Prognosis is typically poor and may represent progression of underlying malignancy [58] (Fig. 10).

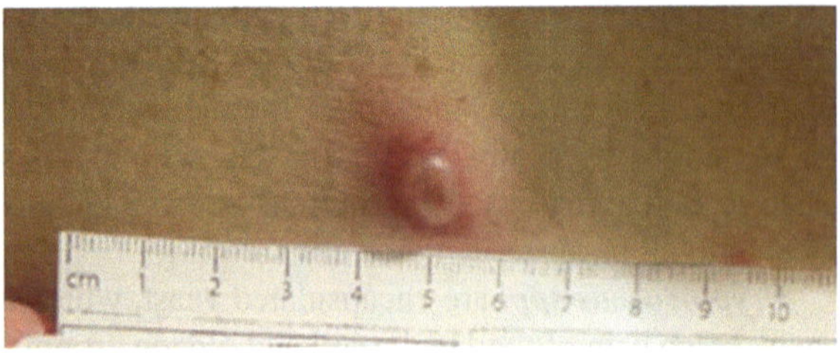

Fig. 10 Skin examination shows a tense bullae with surrounding erythema. Histopathology revealed leukemia cutis in the setting of AML

Sweet's syndrome (Acute Febrile Neutrophilic Dermatosis)

Sweet's syndrome (SS) is characterized by the development of fever, a painful rash, and leukocytosis [58]. SS can occur in the presence of an underlying malignancy such as AML, CML, MDS or myelofibrosis. It is also known to be drug-induced and can occur secondary to infections, classically it is described after an upper respiratory tract infection [60]. The skin lesions are often erythematous or violaceous papules, nodules or plaques which are tender. Vesicles or bullae can develop due to edema of the upper dermis [60]. A unique finding in SS is pathergy. Cutaneous findings may appear after trauma including venipuncture or biopsy [61]. Histopathology shows neutrophilic infiltrates of the dermal papillae without evidence of leukoclastic vasculitis. Unlike leukemia cutis, the neutrophils that infiltrate the dermis are typically mature [60, 62]. When considering SS it is important to rule out an underlying infection; an important differential diagnosis is pyoderma gangrenosum. Treatment of the underlying malignancy is necessary but steroids can also be utilized [63] (Fig. 11).

Pyoderma Gangrenosum

Pyoderma gangrenosum is an ulcerative neutrophilic dermatosis. PG is associated with many inflammatory and autoimmune conditions including both hematologic malignancies and solid tumors [64]. It is typically a diagnosis of exclusion but is characterized by a rapidly developing, painful ulceration with undermined borders. Like Sweet's Syndrome it may exhibit pathergy [65]. The base of the ulcer is typically necrotic with a surrounding erythematous or violaceous halo [66]. The bullous subtype is characterized by bullae formation preceding the ulceration and is commonly associated with hematologic malignancies [58]. Skin biopsy from the border

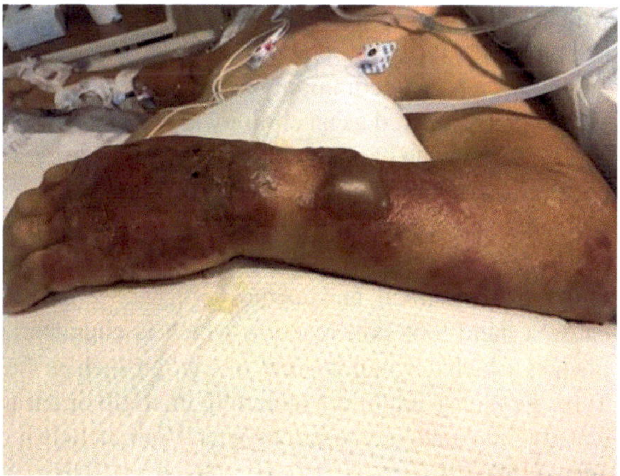

Fig. 11 Erythematous and edematous plaque of the hand with large bullae of the forearm. There are several annular erythematous lesions of the proximal arm. The two round hyperpigmented lesions of the dorsum of the hand represent punch biopsy sites. Histopathology revealed sweet's syndrome in the setting of MDS

of the ulcer should be obtained although it is difficult to diagnose PG based on pathology due to changing histology with the evolution of the ulcer. Examination may reveal dense neutrophilic infiltrates with leukoclastic vasculitis or necrosis [67]. Treatment with steroids usually results in rapid improvement [66].

Vasculitis

Paraneoplastic vasculitis is most commonly associated with MDS and other hematologic malignancies [68]. It is characterized by non-blanchable palpable purpura which may be painful or pruritic [58, 69]. Biopsy is essential for diagnosis and will show necrotizing leukocytoclastic vasculitis with fibrinoid necrosis and neutrophil infiltration of the vessel wall [70]. The presentation of vasculitis may precede the diagnosis of cancer but can also present at all stages of disease [68]. Treatment of the underlying malignancy can result in resolution of the vasculitis [58].

Medication Reactions

Many medications that patients have exposure to during the treatment of malignancies can lead to rashes and skin pathology. It is important to monitor for allergic drug rashes which usually resolve with discontinuation of the inciting medication. Steven-Johnson syndrome (SJS) and toxic epidermal necrolysis (TEN) are both drug reactions that have a high mortality rate due to epidermal sloughing. SJS and TEN may begin with a prodrome which includes high fever. Skin findings may begin with erythematous macules or targetoid lesions progressing to the development of bullae and erosions [71]. Nikolsky sign is often positive. Many patients will also have mucosal involvement [72]. The two conditions are distinguished from each other based on body surface involvement; SJS involves <10% and TEN involves >30% with an overlap of disease characterization between 10–30% [71]. Many drugs have been linked to the development of SJS or TEN, particularly antibiotics. Sulfonamide antibiotics are most commonly associated with SJS or TEN however all antibiotics should be considered as an etiology [71, 73] (Figs. 12 and 13).

Toxic erythema of chemotherapy is a nonallergic reaction that is caused by many chemotherapeutic agents. Toxic erythema of chemotherapy presents with painful erythema and edema which can be present on the hands and feet or intertriginous areas. It is most commonly associated with methotrexate, cytarabine, anthracyclines, 5-fluorouracil, and taxanes [58]. Multikinase inhibitors such as sorafenib can cause a hand-foot-skin reaction which is characterized by painful hyperkeratotic plaques which develop in areas of friction such as the fingertips and joints [58, 74]. Tyrosine kinase inhibitors including imatinib or dasatinib are also commonly associated with cutaneous reactions which can include a maculopapular rash and facial edema [58, 75].

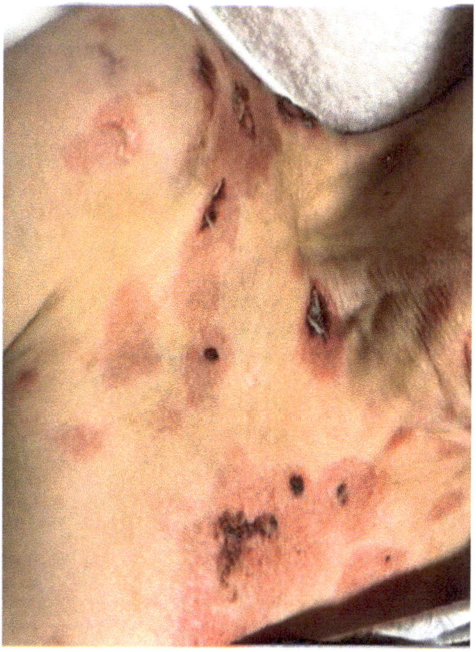

Fig. 12 Cutaneous examination showing erythematous macules with areas of central ulceration consistent with Stevens-Johnson Syndrome in a patient with a history of Burkitt's Lymphoma receiving vancomycin

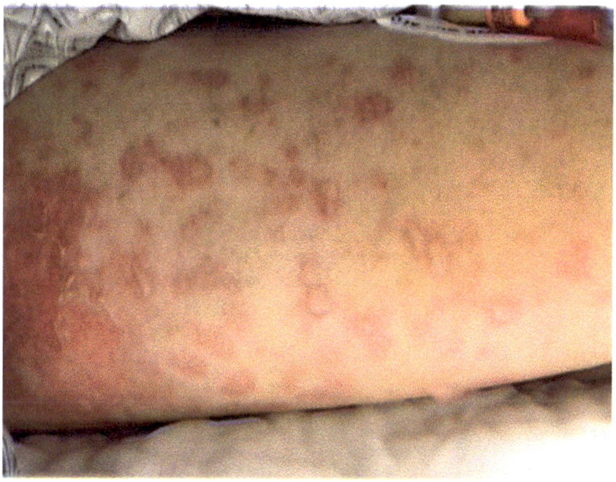

Fig. 13 The above patient in Fig. 12 developed numerous bullae with areas of erosions and sloughing leading to denuded skin consistent with the diagnosis of Stevens-Johnson Syndrome

Key Points

Rash description	Pathogen
Cellulitis	Staphylococcus, Streptococcus including Streptococcus Pneumonia, Bacillus, Clostridium, Corynebacterium JK, Pseudomonas, E.coli, Serratia, Stenotrophomonas, Aeromonas, Chromobacterium. Aspergillus, Fusarium, Candidiasis, Mucormycosis. Non Tuberculous Mycobacteria.

(continued)

Rash description	Pathogen
Pustules	Staphylococcus aureus, Bacillus, Corynebacterium, Gram negative bacteria (mainly Ecoli, Citrobacter, chromobacterium). Mycobacteria. Candidiasis, Histoplasmosis, Aspergillosis, Fusarium. HSV/HZV.
Necrotic Lesion	Pseudomonas, other Gram negative bacilli (mainly E coli, Stenotrophomonas, Citrobacter), Bacillus, Clostridium, Corynebacterium. Aspergillus, Candidiasis, Mucormycosis, Fusarium. HSV/HZV/CMV.
Subcutaneous nodules	Staphylococcus aureus, Corynebacterium JK, Pseudomonas, E coli, Stenotrophomonas. Mycobacteria. Aspergillosis, Fusarium. Candidiasis, Coccidiomycosis, Cryptococcus, Histoplasmosis.
Ulcers	Pseudomonas, other Gram negative bacilli (including but not limited to E coli, Serratia, Stenotrophomonas, Citrobacter, Chromobacterium), Bacillus. Mycobacteria. Aspergillosis, Candidiasis, Mucormycosis, Coccidiomycosis, Histoplasmosis. HSV/HZV/CMV
Vesicle or Bullae	Bacillus cereus, Clostridium, Staphylococcus, Pseudomonas, other gram negative bacilli (Klebsiella, E. coli, Aeromonas, Enterobacter, Stenotrophomonas). Aspergillus, Fusarium. HSV/HZV. Mycobactrium tuberculosis.
Ecthyma gangrenosum	Pseudomonas, E coli, Klebsiella, Morganella, Aeromonas, Serratia, Vibrio, Citrobacter, Stenotrophomonas. Aspergillus, Candidiasis, Mucormycosis, Fusarium [3]
Acral Hemorrhagic Bullae	Clostridium, Streptococcus, Bacillus, Pseudomonas, Citrobacter, Enterobacter, E coli, Klebseilla, Morganella. Aspergillus, Fusarium [3] HSV/HZV [3]

References

1. Kryeziu E, Kryeziu K, Bajraktari G, Abazi M, Zylfiu B, Rudhani I, Sh S, Ukimeri A, Brovina A, Sh D, Telaku S. Ecthyma gangrenosum in a patient with acute leukemia. Med Arh. 2010;64(6):373–4.
2. Brady GP, Bolivar R, Fainstein V, et al. Infections caused by Pseudomonas aeruginosa. Rev Infect Dis. 1983;5:279–313.
3. Grossman ME, Fox LP, Kovarik C, Rosenbach M. Cutaneous manifestations of infection in the immunocompromised host. 2nd ed. New York: Springer Science+Business Media, LLC; 2012. https://doi.org/10.1007/978-1-4419-1578-8.
4. Bodey GP. Dermatologic manifestations of infections in neutropenic patients. Infect Dis Clin N Am. 1994;8(3):655–75. Review.

5. Mull JD, Callahan WS. The role of the elastase of Pseudomonas aeruginosa in experimental infection. Exp Mol Pathol. 1995;4:567–75.
6. Brzozowski D, Ross DC. Upper limb Escherichia coli cellulitis in the immunocompromised. J Hand Surg Br. 1997;22(5):679–80.
7. Livingston W, Grossman ME, Garvey G. Hemorrhagic bullae in association with Enterobacter cloacae septicemia. J Am Acad Dermatol. 1992;27:637–8.
8. Chapman RA, Van Slyck EJ, Madhavan T. Skin lesions associated with E. coli sepsis in a patient with acute leukemia. Henry Ford Hosp Med J. 1980;28(1):47–8.
9. Grant MD, Horowitz HI, Lorian V. Gangrenous ulcer and septicemia due to citrobacter. N Engl J Med. 1969;280(23):1286–7.
10. Gössl M, Eggebrecht H. Necrotizing skin ulceration in antibiotic-induced agranulocytosis. Mayo Clin Proc. 2006;81(12):1527.
11. Sakhnini E, Weissmann A, Oren I. Fulminant Stenotrophomonas maltophilia soft tissue infection in immunocompromised patients: an outbreak transmitted via tap water. Am J Med Sci. 2002;323(5):269–72.
12. Harris RL, Faintein V, Elting L, et al. Bacteremia caused by Aeromonas species hospitalized cancer patients. Rev Infect Dis. 1985;7:314–20.
13. Klastersky J. Infections in immunocompromised patients. I. Pathogenesis, etiology, and diagnosis. Clin Ther. 1985;8(1):90–9.
14. Cone LA, Dreisbach L, Potts BE, Comess BE, Burleigh WA. Fatal Bacillus cereus endocarditis masquerading as an anthrax-like infection in a patient with acute lymphoblastic leukemia: case report. J Heart Valve Dis. 2005;14(1):37–9.
15. Mori T, Tokuhira M, Takae Y, et al. Successful non-surgical treatment of brain abscess and necrotizing fasciitis caused by Bacillus cereus. Intern Med. 2002;41(8):671–3.
16. Groschel D, Burgess MA, Bodey GP. Gas gangrene-like infection with Bacillus cereus in a lymphoma patient. Cancer. 1976;37:988–91.
17. Bodey GP, Rodriguez S, Fainstein V, et al. Clostridial bacteremia in cancer patients. Cancer. 1991;67:1928–42.
18. Hopkins DG, Kushner JP. Clostridial species in the pathogenesis of necrotizing enterocolitis in patients with neutropenia. Am J Hematol. 1983;14:289–95.
19. Van der Lelie H, Leverstein-Van Hall M, Mertens M, et al. Corynebacterium CDC group JK (Corynebacterium jeikeium) sepsis in haematological patients: a report of three cases and a systematic literature review. Scand J Infect Dis. 1995;27(6):581–4.
20. Olson JM, Nguyen VQ, Yoo J, Kuechle MK. Cutaneous manifestations of Corynebacterium jeikeium sepsis. Int J Dermatol. 2009;48(8):886–8.
21. Elting LS, Bodey GP, Keefe BH. Septicemia and shock syndrome due to viridans streptococci: a case – control study of predisposing factors. Clin Infect Dis. 1992;14:1201–7.
22. Van Ingen J. Diagnosis of nontuberculous mycobacterial infections. Semin Respir Crit Care Med. 2013;34(pg):103–9.
23. Roukens AH, Mendels EJ, Verbeet NL, Borne PA v d, Nicolae-Cristea AR, Bentvelsen RG, van Doorn R, de Boer MG. Disseminated cutaneous Mycobacterium chelonae infection in a patient with acute myeloid leukemia. Open Forum Infect Dis. 2014;1(3):ofu103. https://doi.org/10.1093/ofid/ofu103.
24. McWhinney PH, Yates M, Prentice HG, et al. Infection caused by Mycobacterium chelonae: a diagnostic and therapeutic problem in the neutropenic patient, Clin Infect Dis, 1992, vol. 14(pg. 1208–1212).
25. Roukens AH, Mendels EJ, Verbeet NL, et al. Disseminated cutaneous mycobacterium chelonae infection in a patient with acute myeloid leukemia. Open Forum Infect Dis. 2014;1(3):ofu103. https://doi.org/10.1093/ofid/ofu103. Published 2014 Nov 26.
26. Doucette K, Fishman JA. Nontuberculous mycobacterial infection in hematopoietic stem cell and solid organ transplant patients. Clin Infect Dis. 2004;38:1428–39.
27. Doutre MS, Beylot C, Mougein J, et al. Cutaneous infection caused by Mycobacterium malmoense in a patient with myelodysplastic syndrome. J R Soc Med. 1993;86:110–1.

28. Naorungroj S, Aiempanakit K. A study of cutaneous manifestations among febrile neutropenic patients: a five-year retrospective review in a single tertiary university hospital in Southern Thailand. J Am Acad Dermatol. 74(5):AB166. https://doi.org/10.1016/j.jaad.2016.02.653.
29. Feld R, Evans WK, DeBoer G. Herpes zoster in patients with small-cell carcimona of the lung receiving combined modality treatment. Ann Intern Med. 1980;93:282–3.
30. Mays SR, Bogle MA, Bodey GP. Cutaneous fungal infections in the oncology patient: recognition and management. Am J Clin Dermatol. 2006;7(1):31–43.
31. Pappas PG, et al. Clinical practice guideline for the management of candidiasis: 2016 update by the Infectious Diseases Society of America. Clin Infect Dis. 2016;62(4):e1–50.
32. Horn DL, et al. Epidemiology and outcomes of candidemia in 2019 patients: data from the prospective antifungal therapy alliance registry. Clin Infect Dis. 2009;48(12):1695–703.
33. Sipsas NV, et al. Candidemia in patients with hematologic malignancies in the era of new antifungal agents (2001–2007): stable incidence but changing epidemiology of a still frequently lethal infection. Cancer. 2009;115(20):4745–52.
34. Guarana M, Nucci M. Acute disseminated candidiasis with skin lesions: a systematic review. Clin Microbiol Infect. 2018;24(3):246–50.
35. Chen LY, et al. Associated clinical characteristics of patients with candidemia among different Candida species. J Microbiol Immunol Infect. 2013;46(6):463–8.
36. Nucci M, Anaissie E. Cutaneous infection by Fusarium species in healthy and immunocompromised hosts: implications for diagnosis and management. Clin Infect Dis. 2002;35(8):909–20.
37. Nucci M, Anaissie E. Fusarium infections in immunocompromised patients. Clin Microbiol Rev. 2007;20(4):695–704.
38. Hay RJ. Fusarium infections of the skin. Curr Opin Infect Dis. 2007;20(2):115–7.
39. Hayashida MZ, et al. Disseminated fusariosis with cutaneous involvement in hematologic malignancies: report of six cases with high mortality rate. An Bras Dermatol. 2018;93(5):726–9.
40. Gilbert DN, et al., editors. The Sanford guide to antimicrobial therapy 2018. Sperryville: Antimicrobial Therapy, Inc; 2018.
41. Bernardeschi C, et al. Cutaneous invasive aspergillosis: retrospective multicenter study of the French invasive-aspergillosis registry and literature review. Medicine (Baltimore). 2015;94(26):e1018.
42. Patterson TF, et al. Invasive aspergillosis. Disease spectrum, treatment practices, and outcomes. I3 Aspergillus Study Group. Medicine (Baltimore). 2000;79(4):250–60.
43. Branscomb R. An overview of mucormycosis. Lab Med. 2002;33(6):453–5.
44. Patterson TF, et al. Practice guidelines for the diagnosis and management of aspergillosis: 2016 update by the Infectious Diseases Society of America. Clin Infect Dis. 2016;63(4):e1–e60.
45. Petrikkos G, et al. Epidemiology and clinical manifestations of mucormycosis. Clin Infect Dis. 2012;54(Suppl 1):S23–34.
46. Roden MM, et al. Epidemiology and outcome of zygomycosis: a review of 929 reported cases. Clin Infect Dis. 2005;41(5):634–53.
47. Ingram CW, et al. Disseminated zygomycosis: report of four cases and review. Rev Infect Dis. 1989;11(5):741–54.
48. Sun HY, Singh N. Mucormycosis: its contemporary face and management strategies. Lancet Infect Dis. 2011;11(4):301–11.
49. Chang P, Rodas C. Skin lesions in histoplasmosis. Clin Dermatol. 2012;30(6):592–8.
50. Lemos LB, Baliga M, Guo M. Blastomycosis: the great pretender can also be an opportunist. Initial clinical diagnosis and underlying diseases in 123 patients. Ann Diagn Pathol. 2002;6(3):194–203.
51. Miceli A, Krishnamurthy K. Blastomycosis. Treasure Island: StatPearls; 2018.
52. Wang S, et al. Dermatoscopic and clinicopathologic findings of cutaneous blastomycosis. J Am Acad Dermatol. 2015;73(5):e169–70.
53. DiCaudo DJ. Coccidioidomycosis: a review and update. J Am Acad Dermatol. 2006;55(6):929–42; quiz 943–5.
54. Christianson JC, Engber W, Andes D. Primary cutaneous cryptococcosis in immunocompetent and immunocompromised hosts. Med Mycol. 2003;41(3):177–88.

55. Perfect JR, Bicanic T. Cryptococcosis diagnosis and treatment: what do we know now. Fungal Genet Biol. 2015;78:49–54.
56. Grunwald MR, McDonnell MH, Induru R, Gerber JM. Cutaneous manifestations in leukemia patients. Semin Oncol. 2016;43(3):359–65.
57. Kang YS, Kim HS, Park HJ, Lee JY, Kim HO, Cho BK, et al. Clinical characteristics of 75 patients with leukemia cutis. J Korean Med Sci. 2013;28(4):614–9.
58. Li AW, Yin ES, Stahl M, Kim TK, Panse G, Zeidan AM, et al. The skin as a window to the blood: cutaneous manifestations of myeloid malignancies. Blood Rev. 2017;31(6):370–88.
59. Benet C, Gomez A, Aguilar C, Delattre C, Vergier B, Beylot-Barry M, et al. Histologic and immunohistologic characterization of skin localization of myeloid disorders: a study of 173 cases. Am J Clin Pathol. 2011;135(2):278–90.
60. Cohen PR. Sweet's syndromeDOUBLEHYPHENa comprehensive review of an acute febrile neutrophilic dermatosis. Orphanet J Rare Dis. 2007;2:34.
61. Qiao J, Wang Y, Bai J, Wu Y, Fang H. Concurrence of Sweet's syndrome, pathergy phenomenon and erythema nodosum-like lesions. An Bras Dermatol. 2015;90(2):237–9.
62. Going JJ, Going SM, Myskow MW, Beveridge GW. Sweet's syndrome: histological and immunohistochemical study of 15 cases. J Clin Pathol. 1987;40(2):175–9.
63. Paydas S. Sweet's syndrome: a revisit for hematologists and oncologists. Crit Rev Oncol Hematol. 2013;86(1):85–95.
64. Kridin K, Cohen AD, Amber KT. Underlying systemic diseases in pyoderma Gangrenosum: a systematic review and meta-analysis. Am J Clin Dermatol. 2018;19(4):479–87.
65. Braswell SF, Kostopoulos TC, Ortega-Loayza AG. Pathophysiology of pyoderma gangrenosum (PG): an updated review. J Am Acad Dermatol. 2015;73(4):691–8.
66. Su WP, Davis MD, Weenig RH, Powell FC, Perry HO. Pyoderma gangrenosum: clinicopathologic correlation and proposed diagnostic criteria. Int J Dermatol. 2004;43(11):790–800.
67. Crowson AN, Mihm MC Jr, Magro C. Pyoderma gangrenosum: a review. J Cutan Pathol. 2003;30(2):97–107.
68. Loricera J, Calvo-Rio V, Ortiz-Sanjuan F, Gonzalez-Lopez MA, Fernandez-Llaca H, Rueda-Gotor J, et al. The spectrum of paraneoplastic cutaneous vasculitis in a defined population: incidence and clinical features. Medicine (Baltimore). 2013;92(6):331–43.
69. Greer JM, Longley S, Edwards NL, Elfenbein GJ, Panush RS. Vasculitis associated with malignancy. Experience with 13 patients and literature review. Medicine (Baltimore). 1988;67(4):220–30.
70. Garcia-Porrua C, Gonzalez-Gay MA. Cutaneous vasculitis as a paraneoplastic syndrome in adults. Arthritis Rheum. 1998;41(6):1133–5.
71. Miliszewski MA, Kirchhof MG, Sikora S, Papp A, Dutz JP. Stevens-Johnson syndrome and toxic epidermal necrolysis: an analysis of triggers and implications for improving prevention. Am J Med. 2016;129(11):1221–5.
72. Schwartz RA, McDonough PH, Lee BW. Toxic epidermal necrolysis: part I. Introduction, history, classification, clinical features, systemic manifestations, etiology, and immunopathogenesis. J Am Acad Dermatol. 2013;69(2):173, e1–13; quiz 85–6.
73. Roujeau JC, Kelly JP, Naldi L, Rzany B, Stern RS, Anderson T, et al. Medication use and the risk of Stevens-Johnson syndrome or toxic epidermal necrolysis. N Engl J Med. 1995;333(24):1600–7.
74. Macdonald JB, Macdonald B, Golitz LE, LoRusso P, Sekulic A. Cutaneous adverse effects of targeted therapies: part I: inhibitors of the cellular membrane. J Am Acad Dermatol. 2015;72(2):203–18; quiz 19–20.
75. Brazzelli V, Grasso V, Borroni G. Imatinib, dasatinib and nilotinib: a review of adverse cutaneous reactions with emphasis on our clinical experience. J Eur Acad Dermatol Venereol. 2013;27(12):1471–80.

Bacteremia in Neutropenic Patients

Sheila Hernandez, Ana Paula Velez, Jorge Lamarche, and John N. Greene

Abstract Neutropenic patients are predisposed to polymicrobial infections that may cause substantial morbidity and mortality. Neutropenia is defined as a neutrophil count of <500 cells/mm^3, or a count of <1000 cells/mm^3 with a predicted decrease to <500 cells/mm^3. Many factors play a role in the development of bacteremia such as the use of cytotoxic chemotherapy that leads to neutropenia, and also contributes to the disruption of skin and mucosal barriers. Moreover, exposure to pathogens is possible due to the frequent utilization of foley catheters and venous catheters in patients with cancer (Rolston et al., Clin Infect Dis 45(2):228–233, 2007). Lastly, the use of prophylactic antibiotics can lead to breakthrough MDR bacteria limiting antimicrobial options for therapy (Rolston et al., Clin Infect Dis 45(2):228–233, 2007; Perez et al., Clin Infect Dis 59(Suppl 5):S335–S339, 2014).

Both gram-negative and gram-positive organisms are culpable for infection in these immunocompromised patients. Although gram-negative bacteremia is still a leading cause in most recent years, infections by gram-positive bacteria have increased. This could be secondary to the wide use of long-term vascular catheters (Holland et al., Clin Infect Dis 59(Suppl 5):S331–S334, 2014; Baskaran et al., Int J Infect Dis: IJID: Off Publ Int Soc Infect Dis 11(6):513–517, 2007).

The most common microorganisms that cause bacteremia in neutropenic patients are the Enterobacteracie group, *Pseudomonas aeruginosa*, *Staphylococcus aureus*, Coagulase negative *Staphylococci*, and *streptococcus species*. In addition, other species will be discussed in this chapter (Rolston et al., Clin Infect Dis 45(2):228–

S. Hernandez, MD
International Scholar at Moffitt Cancer Center, Tampa, FL, USA

A. P. Velez, MD, FACP (✉)
Associate Professor, University of South Florida, Tampa, FL, USA
e-mail: ana.velez@moffitt.org

J. Lamarche, MD
USF Morsani College of Medicine James Haley VA Hospital, James Haley VA Hospital, Tampa, FL, USA

J. N. Greene, MD, FACP
USF Morsani College of Medicine, Moffitt Cancer Center and Research Institute, Tampa, FL, USA

A. P. Velez et al. (eds.), *Infections in Neutropenic Cancer Patients*,
https://doi.org/10.1007/978-3-030-21859-1_6

233, 2007; Baskaran et al., Int J Infect Dis: IJID: Off Publ Int Soc Infect Dis 11(6):513–517, 2007; Yadegarynia et al., Caspian J Int Med 4(3):698–701, 2013).

Less common bacteria including nocardia and *mycobacterium spp* will not be discussed in this chapter.

Keywords Viridans Group Streptococci (VGS) · Toxic shock-like syndrome · Stenotrophomona Maltophilia · VRE colonization · C. jeikeium · Rothia mucilaginosa · Fusobacterium necrophorum · F. nucleatum · Carbapenemase-producing Klebsiella pneumoniae (KPC) · Pseudomonas aeruginosa · MRSA · Multidrug resistant (MDR)

Gram Positive Organisms

Gram positive bacteria have been an important cause of bacteremia in neutropenic patients. Many studies have concluded that this rate is only increasing exponentially over the years. One study from the International Antimicrobial Therapy Cooperative Group of the European Organization for Research and Treatment of Cancer documented that almost 30% of single microorganism isolates recovered during mid 1970's were Gram positive bacteria, compared with 67% of such organisms isolated during the early 1990's [1]. Among the most common organisms are *Staphylococcus aureus*, coagulase negative *Staphylococcus* and *streptococcus* species. A very important cause of bacteremia in patients with neutropenia and cancer is Viridans group streptococci (VGS), originating from the normal flora in humans [1].

Viridans Group Streptoccoci (VGS)

In most recent years, the isolation of VGS from the blood of neutropenic patients with cancer has increased. *Streptococcus mitis* has been the most common pathogen in these cases. VGS are part of the oral cavity flora. They are also found on the skin, female genital tract, upper respiratory tract and the gastrointestinal tract. In normal conditions this organism has low morbidity, but they cause serious infection when the oral mucosa or other sites are compromised along with a deficient host defense such as in a patient with neutropenia and cancer.

In neutropenic patients, this organism can cause very high fevers for several days in spite of proper antibiotics. In addition, it has been associated with toxic shock like syndrome and ARDS as discussed below.

Severe neutropenia is an important factor for VGS bacteremia. Other risk factors include bone marrow transplantation and mucositis [2].

Chemotherapy induced gastric ulcers may allow streptococci to grow in an environment with low acid protection due to the administration of agents such as proton pump inhibitors, histamine 2 blockers and antacids [1].

Chemotherapeutic agents predispose the patients to immunosupression. Cytosine arabinoside, which is an antimetabolic agent used in the treatment of acute myeloid leukemia, acute lymphocytic leukemia and lymphomas, at high doses has been implicated as a risk factor for bacteremia with VGS. Certain antimicrobial agents may predispose to bacteremia with VGS. Oral prophylaxis with either sulfamethoxazole trimethoprin or fluoroquinolones has been highly associated with VGS due to the resistance of this bacteria to these agents [3, 4].

Viridans Streptococci Toxic Shock-like Syndrome and ARDS

In approximately 21–25% of children post- bone marrow transplant, a toxic shock-like syndrome has been reported with VGS bacteremia. The usual organism isolated is *S. mitis*. This syndrome is very rare in patients without neutropenia and presents with hypotension, palmar desquamation, respiratory distress syndrome, rash, fever, and confusion, which can rapidly progress to coma, multiple organ failure and death. This syndrome usually occurs within 2 or 3 days after presentation. The symptoms may worsen and produce respiratory symptoms within 48 h. This complication is believed to be immunologically mediated [5].

ARDS presents with hypoxia and shortness of breath. Cough and fever are often present. Tachycardia and tachypnea are common features and may be the initial symptoms. Occasionally, patients may experience pleuritic pain followed by hypoxia and respiratory failure [6].

Resistance of VGS against many antibiotics has been increasingly recognized. In early studies, it was concluded that this pathogen was susceptible to penicillin, however, some studies have described intermediate and high-level penicillin resistance. Resistances against second generation cephalosporins, such as Cefuroxime and third generation cephalosporins like Ceftriaxone have also been described [1].

Due to its high efficacy and low resistance, Vancomycin is routinely given in addition to various β-lactam agents (cefepime, ceftriaxone, piperacillin tazobactam or carbapenem) as part of the initial empirical antimicrobial regimens for neutropenic patients with VGS bacteremia [1] (Table 1). Once susceptibilities results are available, vancomycin can be discontinued if indicated.

If hypoxia is present, corticostisteroids should be given to prevent the development of ARDS and respiratory failure [5].

The mortality rate due to VGS bacteremia in spite of appropriate antibiotics can fluctuate from 0 to 20% but can increase up to 60–100%if toxic shock like syndrome develops [1].

Staphylococcus aureus

S. aureus is a major cause of infection in neutropenic patients with cancer. Although *S. aureus* is most commonly implicated in soft tissue infections and pneumonia, it is responsible for almost 15% of bacteremia cases [7].

Table 1 Gram positive organisms bacteremia

Gram positive cocci	**Therapy**
Viridans Strepotococci	Ceftriaxone, cefepime, piperacillin tazobactam, or carbapenem plus vancomycin until susceptibilities are available
Methicillin sensitive *Staphylococcus aureus*	Nafcillin, oxacillin or cefazolin
Methicillin resistant *Staphylococcus aureus*	Vancomycin or daptomycin
Vancomycin sensitive Enterococci	Ampicillin, piperacillin or vancomycin
Vancomycin resistant *Enterococci*	Daptomycin, or linezolid
Rothia mucilaginosa (coco-bacilli)	Vancomycin until susceptibilities are available, then may de-escalate to beta-lactam depending on susceptibilities
Gram positive rods	**Therapy**
Corynebacterium species	Vancomycin
Lactobacillus	Penicillin, ampicillin, piperacillin, or clindamycin

The presence of pneumonia and bacteremia results in a mortality rate for up to 50% which is higher than that observed in patients without cancer.

Treatment of *S. aureus* bacteremia in neutropenic patients does not differ from the non-neutropenic. Early removal of the central venous catheter (CVC) and prolonged intravenous antibiotic therapy for several weeks is recommended especially for complicated endovascular infections and persistent bacteremias [8, 9].

Initial empiric treatment should include vancomycin until methicillin resistant *Staphylococcus aureus* (MRSA) is excluded. If methicillin sensitive *Staphylococcus* is isolated, vancomycin can be de-escalated to a beta-lactam agent such as nafcillin, oxacillin, or cefazolin (Table 1).

Echocardiogram is recommended for all the patients with *S. aureus* bacteremia to rule out endocarditis [10, 11].

Enterococci

Enterococci spp are low virulence organisms; however, they represent a major cause of bacteremia in the cancer population. *E. faecalis* and *E. faecium* are the most common species of enterococcus bacteremia in cancer patients. Risk factors for bacteremia include nosocomial infection, prior antibiotic exposure including levofloxacin, prolonged neutropenia, and stem cell transplantation [12, 13].

Enterococci faecium susceptibilities to B-Lactam antibiotics varies, and vancomycin resistance is increasing [14].

The mechanism of resistance of Vancomycin-resistant enterococci (VRE) is due to the change in the bacterial cell wall decreasing the affinity of vancomycin to its site of action. VRE species more commonly encode the *VanA* and the *VanB* genotypes followed by the *VanD* and the *VanC* genotypes [15].

Colonization of VRE in the stool of neutropenic patients, represent high risk of subsequent VRE bacteremia [13, 16].

The treatment of choice for enterococcus bacteremia includes penicillin type of antibiotics such as ampicillin or piperacillin provided that the organism is sensitive. Vancomycin is also an option for penicillin allergic patients (Table 1). Compared with other streptococcus species, enterococcus are more resistant to killing by monotherapy with the above antibiotics. Combination therapy including aminoglycosides or double beta lactam including ceftriaxone is usually recommended for endocarditis. Data on combination therapy for uncomplicated enterococcus bacteremia are scarce.

Daptomycin and linezolid are the most widely used antibiotics for VRE *faecium* or VRE *fecalis* bacteremia [15] (Table 1).

In vitro studies have revealed synergy when using daptomycin in combination with ampicillin or ceftaroline for complicated and persistent VRE bacteremia [17].

Corynebacterium

Corynebacterium are aerobic, gram positive, catalase-positive, nonsporulating, nonmotile rods. There are many subtypes of Corynebacterium, such as *C. diptheriae* and nondiptherial, like *Corynebaterium striatum*, *Corynebacterium amycolatum*, *Corynebacterium minutissimum*, *Corynebacterium xerosis*, *Corynebacterium freneyi* and *Corynebacterium jeikeium*. They were thought to be contaminants as they are present in the normal flora, but recent studies have shown that they are opportunistic pathogens in immunocompromised hosts with cancer and hematologic malignancies. In this section, we will review the Corynebactrerium species most relevant in neutropenic patients.

Corynebacterium striatum

Corynebacterium striatum colonize the skin and mucous membranes of humans. They are also found in the environment. *C. striatum* has rarely been reported to be a pathogen, causing pulmonary infections and bacteremia only in immunocompromised patients. Infections are also associated with implanted indwelling devices. Thrombophlebitis associated with central venous catheters has been reported. The majority of *C. Striatum* infections are nosocomial wound infections and less often, systemic infections.

All strains of *C. striatum* are resistant to penicillin, but are susceptible to other beta lactam antibiotics and to vancomycin. For serious infections vancomycin is the drug of choice [18, 19] (Table 1).

Corynebacterium jeikeium

C. jeikeium is only pathogenic for humans. It is found in soil and water and is part of normal human skin flora. The colonization rate increases with hospitalization. *C. jeikeium* is the most common cause of diphtheroid endocarditis of prosthetic valves.

C. jeikeium infections may present with skin and soft tissue lesions in patients who are granulocytopenic. Lesions are usually at local infection sites of previous bone marrow biopsy, intravascular catheter insertion, or perianal fissures. The lesions usually precede septicemia and are designated as the primary source of infection [20, 21].

Corynebacterium jeikeium is highly resistant to beta-lactam agents, aminoglycosides, and quinolones. Vancomycin is the most active antibiotic (Table 1). High level daptomycin resistance is rare with one case report of bacteremia reported [22].

In general, removal of the CVC is recommended in order to clear the bacteremia. Removal of involved prosthetic device is usually required for cure [22].

Rothia mucilaginosa

Rothia mucilaginosa (previously known *Stomatococcus mucilaginosus*) is an aerobic or facultative anaerobic gram positive cocco bacilli. *Rothia spp* are part of the oropharynx flora and can be associated with periodontal disease. Risk factors for invasive disease include profound neutropenia, alcoholism, liver disease and HIV infection. Clinical syndromes include bacteremia, endocarditis, meningitis, pneumonia, and infections of the bone and soft tissues [23].

Previous studies have demonstrated that *Rothia spp* are susceptible to most beta lactam agents, however species with partial resistance to penicillin and methicillin have been recently described. Given concerns for beta lactam resistace, vancomycin is the ideal empiric therapy for *Rothia mucilaginosa* bacteremia until susceptibilities are available [23] (Table 1).

Lactobacillus

Lactobacilli are gram positive microareophilic organisms that are part of the normal oral, gastrointestinal and genitourinary flora. Bacteremia is rare, but the most common species associated with this entity are *Lactobacillus casei* and *Lactobacillus rhamnosus*. Clinical manifestations of Lactobacillus bacteremia can range from asymptomatic to fever, leukocytosis and rigors or severe septicemia and may be combined with pneumonia, deep abdominal abscesses or endocarditis. Some findings also include elevated c – reactive protein values. The infection may be underdiagnosed, because lactobacilli are difficult to culture and to identify and are often confused as contaminants. *L. rhamnosus* cause more severe infections with a higher inflammatory response.

Risk factors include persistent prolonged neutropenia, use of broad-spectrum antibotics, especially vancomycin (which results in the persistence of vancomycin resitant GI flora), corticosteroids and a history of organ transplantation and other immunosuppressive conditions [24].

The treatment of choice for Lactobacillus bacteremia include penicillin, ampicillin and piperacillin. Clindamycin is also an active agent (Table 1). Susceptibilities to cephalosporins varies. Combination therapy with penicillin and aminoglycosides may be required for complicated infections. Lactobacillus are uniformly resistant to vancomycin [25].

Anaerobic Bacteremia

Information on anaerobic bacteremia in cancer patients is very limited since it only represents about 5–9% of all episodes of bacteremia in hospitalized patients. Anaerobic bacteremia may be undetected due to subtle clinical symptoms. Chemotherapy causes mucosal and visceral damage thus increasing the risk of bacteremia related to endogenous anaerobes.

Gastrointestinal and hematological malignancies are the most common underlying diseases, female genital tract malignancies are also important to note. Most cases of anaerobic bacteremia are caused by *Bacteroides fragilis*, *Clostridium perfringens* and *Peptostreptococcus* spp. Other less common pathogens, but still important in neutropenic patients is *Fusobacterium spp.* [26, 27].

Empirical antimicrobial therapy should be started as soon as the infection is suspected. Prompt and adequate therapy is associated with increased survival. In general aminopenicilins, with or without B-lactamase inhibitors, Carbapenems, Clindamycin and Metronidazole are active against anaerobic isolates with some spectrum difference depending on the species isolated [28].

Fusobacterium necrophorum

Fusobacterium necrophorum represents less than 1% of bacteremias in humans. Only a few hundred cases have been reported in the literature. *F. Necrophorum* is associated with severe septicemia also known as necrobacillosis, postanginal sepsis or Lemierre's syndrome.

Lemierre's Syndrome

Lemierre's syndrome is a very serious complication of pharyngeal infection due to *F. necrophorum*. It usually occurs a few days after the onset of a sore throat.

A more concise definition for Lemierre's syndrome is the presence of a history of angina illness or similar clinical findings, followed by internal jugular vein thrombophlebitis which propagates from the tonsillar veins to the internal jugular vein causing septicemia. This causes septic emboli including necrotic abscesses the lungs and other sites such as bones, liver and joints. Isolation of *F. necrophorum* from blood culture or any other sterile site is a good indicator for diagnosis, but it is not found in all cases of this disease. It is not clear whether it is due to external factors such as timing of sampling, prior antibiotic therapy or the association of this disease with other organisms such as Peptostreptococcus.

The diagnosis of Lemierre's syndrome is clinical. Although this is a very rare disease, its peculiar symptoms should prompt clinical suspicion. The onset of rigors 4–12 days after the resolution of the sore throat is classic. The occurrence of chills indicate that the organisms are present in the circulation. Patients may complain of neck pain and tenderness. Anterior cervical lymphadenopathy is often present. Edema at the angle of the jaw, reflecting the development of internal jugular thrombophlebitis may be mistaken for tender cervical nodes [29, 30].

Fusobacterium nucleatum

This Gram-negative bacilli is commonly found in the gastrointestinal, oropharyngeal and respiratory tracts. It is a common cause of periodontal infection. The most common source of bacteremia associated with *F. nucleatum* comes from an oropharyngeal source of infection [31].

Certain risk factors overlap amongst patients with *F. nucleatum* and *F. necrophorum*. The most common types of malignancy associated with bacteremia include lymphoma and acute leukemia. Treatment with intensive chemotherapy, corticosteroids and bone marrow transplantation also increases the risk for bacteremia. Severe oral mucositis caused by chemotherapy is also an important risk factor as it can serve as a portal of entry for a systemic infection and the propagation of a polymicrobial infection with other pathogens, such as Staphylococcus and *E. coli*. Prophylactic treatment with macrolides, especially erythromycin is an important risk factor for *F. necrophorum* infection due to its high resistance [32].

Penicillin, piperacillin-tazobactam, carbapenems, clindamycin and metronidazole are all active against *F. nucleatum F. necrophorum*. [33] (Table 2)

Table 2 Anaerobes bacteremia

Organism	Therapy
Fusobacterium species	Ampicillin sulbactam, piperacillin-tazobactam, carbapenems, metronidazole, clindamycin

Gram-Negative Rods

Gram negative bacilli are a very common cause of bacteremia in neutropenic patients. The most common gram-negative rods causing bacteremia are *Escherichia coli, Klebsiella spp.* and *Pseudomona aeruginosa.* Before the introduction of the antibiotic era, mortality rates in neutropenic patients with leukemia and Gram-negative infections were as high as 91%. In general, Gram-negative bacteria are reported as MDR if not susceptible to at least 3 of the following antimicrobials: Antipseudomonal penicillins, cephalosporins, carbapenems, aminoglycosides or fluorquinolones [34].

In this chapter, we will discuss the most common gram negative organisms that cause bacteremia in neutropenic patients.

Escherichia coli

Escherichia coli is of great concern in immunocompromised patients. There has been an emergence of a resistant *E. coli* sequence type ST131. This type of *E. coli* produces extended-spectrum β-lactamases, and almost all are resistant to fluoroquinolones. Data suggests that this strains of *E. coli* may be the main explanation for the recent increase in antimicrobial resistance. Serious extra-intestinal infections with this Multi Drug Resistant *E. coli* ST131 often leave physicians with limited treatment options, higher costs, and increased usage of last resort antimicrobials, such as carbapenems. *E. coli* is a major pathogen and one of the most common cause of gram negative bacteremia resulting in extended hospital stays. *E. coli*, like many Gram-negative pathogens can cause septic shock with a fatal outcome.

The most common risk factors for *E. coli* bacteremia are solid tumors of the gastrointestinal tract, previous chemotherapy, prior surgery within 10 days and vascular catheter insertion [35–37].

The treatment of choice for *E coli* bacteremia include piperacillin tazobactam, cephalosporins, and carbapenems. Combination with aminoglycosides until susceptibilities are available may be required depending on prior cultures, recent use of antibiotics or local susceptibility data (Table 3).

Klebsiella pneumoniae

Some strains of *Klebsiella pneumonia* are part of the gastrointestinal flora. When the mucosal barrier of the gastrointestinal tract is disrupted, this bacteria can gain access to the blood stream causing serious blood stream infections. Profound neutropenia especially with chemotherapy treatment within 1 month represent a substantial risk for bacteremia [38].

Table 3 gram negative rods bacteremia

Organism	Therapy
Echerichia coli	Piperacillin tazobactam, cephalosporins, or carbapenems. May use combination with aminoglycosides until susceptibilities are available
Klebsiella pneumoniae	Piperacillin tazobactam, cephalosporins, or carbapenems. May use combination with aminoglycosides until susceptibilities are available
Pseudomonas aeruginosa	Piperacillin tazobactam, cefepime, ceftazidime, meropenem, imipenem, doripenem depending on susceptibilities. May use combination with aminoglycosides until susceptibilities are available
Stenotrophomona Maltophila	Sulfamethoxazole-Trimethoprin, minocycline, moxifloxacin

Carbapenemase-producing *Klebsiella pneumoniae* (KPC) has been identified as an important strain causing nosocomial bacteremia in patients with hematologic malignancies and aplastic anemia [39].

Mortality rates for Klebisella bacteremia is higher when the initial empiric treatment is inadequate [40]. Age plays an important role where newborns and elderly are primarily susceptible.

The treatment of choice for klebsiella bacteremia include piperacillin tazobactam, cephalosporins, and carbapenems. Aminoglycosides in combination with the one of the above also can be used for initial empiric therapy pending susceptibilities (Table 3).

Carbapenems are preferable to piperacillin/tazobactam or cephalosporins when a critically ill patient is in need of empirical therapy especially when there is concern for resistance. Patients who receive a carbapenem as monotherapy or combination therapy during the first days after a blood culture is positive for an extended spectrum beta-lacatamse (ESBL) producing *K. pneumoniae,* had a significantly lower mortality than those who received non-carbapenem antibiotics [40].

Pseudomonas aeruginosa

Pseudomonas aeruginosa infections in neutropenic cancer patients have decreased after the implementation of antibiotics with-anti-pseudomonal activity; however, they are still one of the most common gram-negative bacterial species associated in neutropenic patients.

Mortality due to this pathogen is reported to be about 20% and this number can increase in patients receiving inappropriate antibacterial treatment. Polymicrobial infection is associated with a worse prognosis.

Patients with Pseudomonas bacteremia treated with combination empirical antimicrobial therapy prior to the result susceptibility testing are available have a better 30-day survival compared to monotherapy. However, combination antimicrobial therapy given as definitive treatment for *P. aeruginosa* bacteremia does not improve the rate of survival compared to appropriate definitive monotherapy. A potential advantage of initial empiric combination antimicrobial therapy over monotherapy is the higher probability that the infecting pathogen will be covered by at least one of the components of the regimen until susceptibly data is available. Furthermore, different mechanisms of action between two antibiotics may be synergistic, resulting in enhanced bacterial kill activity compared to the additive activities of the antibiotics when assessed separately. Finally, use of combination therapy may suppress emergence of resistant subpopulations of bacteria.

Treatment of pseudomonas bacteremia include piperacillin tazobactam, cefepime, cefazidime, meropenem, imipenem, or doripenem. Aminoglycoside combination therapy may be helpful to broaden the antimicrobial coverage for MDR strains and consequently improve the outcomes of patients with *P. aeruginosa* bacteremia. Once more information is obtained from the cultures, a targeted antimicrobial agent based on the antibiotic susceptibility results may be pursued [41–44] (Table 3).

For more resistant strains of pseudomonas, ceftolozane-tazobactam can be an option [45].

Stenotrophomona Maltophilia

Stenotrophomona Maltophilia is rarely responsible for community-acquired serious infections. Rather, it is usually a commensal, a colonizer, or part of the endogenous flora of hospitalized patients. It has been increasingly reported as a cause of life-threatening infections, especially in the immunocompromised, such as those with hematological malignancy and in recipients of hematopoietic stem cell transplantation (HSCT), indwelling venous catheterization, long-term hospitalization, aggressive chemotherapy and use of broad-spectrum antibiotics including carbapenems [46].

S. maltophilia bacteremia in patients with hematologic malignancies is a serious complication of profound, persistent neutropenia and broad-spectrum antibiotic use. This pathogen is highly resistant and its antimicrobial resistance may increase when patients are treated with antibiotics over extended periods. Inappropriate antibiotic use is associated with an elevated morbidity and mortality [47, 48].

Complications of *S. maltophilia* infections are septic shock, respiratory failure, pulmonary hemorrhage and septic thrombophlebitis. Morbidity and mortality are high; however, the prognosis may be improved by prompt administration of active antibiotics.

S. maltophilia strains are resistant to the majority of agents used for the empirical treatment of febrile neutropenia including most beta-lactams. Sulfamethoxazole-Trimethoprin and minocycline are very active against most stenotrophomona infections [49, 50] (Table 3).

Newer quinolones, particularly in combination with Sulfamethoxazole-Trimethoprin may be an option. Other combination agents can be used depending on the susceptibilities of the organisms [51].

Multidrug Resistant Gram Negative

The widespread use of antibiotics and the emergence of multidrug resistant (MDR) bacteria has shown to increase mortality particularly in immunosuppressed patients. Screening for MDR bacteria may facilitate prompt isolation and directed treatment targeting the MDR bacteria when the patient demonstrates early signs of infection [52].

Carpapenem-Resistant Enterobacteria (CRE)

Neutropenic patients are at risk for enteric gram negative rod bacteremia from gastrointestinal tract translocation. Beta- lactam agents are recommended for empiric therapy of neutropenic fever, however over the last decade, CRE have emerged as a threat particularly to this vulnerable population.

Identification of CRE usually takes up to 3 days using conventional culture methods. This can delay proper treatment significantly increasing mortality [53].

CRE are universally resistant to all beta-lactam agents due to different carbapenemases. Carbapenemase are classified as type A, B, C and D depending on their molecular structure.

The most clinically significant and the most common type in United States is the Class A beta-lactamase known as *klebsiella pneumonia* carbapenemase (KPC) [54].

Class B beta-lactamase are also known as the metallo-beta-lactamases (MBLs). The New Delhi metallo-beta-lactamase is the most clinically significant of this group [55].

Class D beta-lactamases are also named the OXA type enzymes because of their preference to hydrolyze oxacillin over penicillin. Six subgroups have been identify with different degrees of carbapenem hydrolyzing activity [56].

Treatment recommendations for CRE infections is limited and controversial depending on the subtype and susceptibility results. For KPC, ceftazidime-avibactam or meropenem varbobactam are an option provided that the organism is susceptible [57, 58].

Other alternatives particularly for subtypes resistant to the above antimicrobials i.e. the MBLs include a polymyxin based regimen combined with prolonged carbapenem infusion. For polymyxin resistant strains ceftazidime-avibactam in combination with aztreonam has been used [59].

Other antibiotics with a broader spectrum to treat MDR gram negative rods are under different stages of development including imipenem/cilastin with relebactam, avibactam combined with aztreonam or ceftaroline [60].

Newer antibiotics hopefully will offer a light of cure of MDR gram negative infections in neutropenic patients while receiving aggressive chemotherapy.

References

1. Tunkel AR, Sepkowitz KA. Infections caused by viridans streptococci in patients with neutropenia. Clin Infect Dis. 2002;34(11):1524–9.
2. Husain E, Whitehead S, Castell A, Thomas EE, Speert DP. Viridans streptococci bacteremia in children with malignancy: relevance of species identification and penicillin susceptibility. Pediatr Infect Dis J. 2005;24(6):563–6.
3. Wisplinghoff H, Reinert RR, Cornely O, Seifert H. Molecular relationships and antimicrobial susceptibilities of viridans group streptococci isolated from blood of neutropenic cancer patients. J Clin Microbiol. 1999;37(6):1876–80.
4. Razonable RR, Litzow MR, Khaliq Y, Piper KE, Rouse MS, Patel R. Bacteremia due to viridans group Streptococci with diminished susceptibility to Levofloxacin among neutropenic patients receiving levofloxacin prophylaxis. Clin Infect Dis. 2002;34(11):1469–74.
5. Dompeling EC, Donnelly JP, Raemaekers JM, De Pauw BE. Pre-emptive administration of corticosteroids prevents the development of ARDS associated with Streptococcus mitis bacteremia following chemotherapy with high-dose cytarabine. Ann Hematol. 1994;69(2):69–71.
6. Mokart D, van Craenenbroeck T, Lambert J, Textoris J, Brun JP, Sannini A, et al. Prognosis of acute respiratory distress syndrome in neutropenic cancer patients. Eur Respir J. 2012;40(1):169–76.
7. Tong SY, Davis JS, Eichenberger E, Holland TL, Fowler VG Jr. Staphylococcus aureus infections: epidemiology, pathophysiology, clinical manifestations, and management. Clin Microbiol Rev. 2015;28(3):603–61.
8. El Zakhem A, Chaftari AM, Bahu R, El Helou G, Shelburne S, Jiang Y, et al. Central line-associated bloodstream infections caused by Staphylococcus aureus in cancer patients: clinical outcome and management. Ann Med. 2014;46(3):163–8.
9. Ghanem GA, Boktour M, Warneke C, Pham-Williams T, Kassis C, Bahna P, et al. Catheter-related Staphylococcus aureus bacteremia in cancer patients: high rate of complications with therapeutic implications. Medicine. 2007;86(1):54–60.
10. Liu C, Bayer A, Cosgrove SE, Daum RS, Fridkin SK, Gorwitz RJ, et al. Clinical practice guidelines by the infectious diseases society of america for the treatment of methicillin-resistant Staphylococcus aureus infections in adults and children. Clin Infect Dis. 2011;52(3):e18–55.
11. Holland TL, Arnold C, Fowler VG Jr. Clinical management of Staphylococcus aureus bacteremia: a review. JAMA. 2014;312(13):1330–41.
12. Garsin DA, Frank KL, Silanpaa J, Ausubel FM, Hartke A, Shankar N, et al. Pathogenesis and models of enterococcal infection. In: Gilmore MS, Clewell DB, Ike Y, Shankar N, editors. Enterococci: from commensals to leading causes of drug resistant infection. Boston: Massachusetts Eye and Ear Infirmary; 2014.
13. Sanchez-Diaz AM, Cuartero C, Rodriguez JD, Lozano S, Alonso JM, Rodriguez-Dominguez M, et al. The rise of ampicillin-resistant Enterococcus faecium high-risk clones as a frequent intestinal colonizer in oncohaematological neutropenic patients on levofloxacin prophylaxis: a risk for bacteraemia? Clin Microbiol Infect: Off Publ Eur Soc Clin Microbiol Infect Dis. 2016;22(1):59.e1–8.
14. Cetinkaya Y, Falk P, Mayhall CG. Vancomycin-resistant enterococci. Clin Microbiol Rev. 2000;13(4):686–707.
15. Levitus M, Perera TB. Vancomycin-Resistant Enterococci (VRE). StatPearls. Treasure Island: StatPearls Publishing StatPearls Publishing LLC.; 2018.
16. Alevizakos M, Gaitanidis A, Nasioudis D, Tori K, Flokas ME, Mylonakis E. Colonization with vancomycin-resistant enterococci and risk for bloodstream infection among patients with malignancy: a systematic review and meta-analysis. Open Forum Infect Dis. 2017;4(1):ofw246.
17. Bartash R, Nori P. Beta-lactam combination therapy for the treatment of Staphylococcus aureus and Enterococcus species bacteremia: a summary and appraisal of the evidence. Int J Infect Dis: IJID: Off Publ Int Soc Infect Dis. 2017;63:7–12.

18. Daisuke U, Oishi T, Yamane K, Terada K. Corynebacterium striatum bacteremia associated with a catheter-related blood stream infection. Case Rep Infect Dis. 2017;2017:2682149.
19. Watkins DA, Chahine A, Creger RJ, Jacobs MR, Lazarus HM. Corynebacterium striatum: a diphtheroid with pathogenic potential. Clin Infect Dis. 1993;17(1):21–5.
20. Rozdzinski E, Kern W, Schmeiser T, Kurrle E. Corynebacterium jeikeium bacteremia at a tertiary care center. Infection. 1991;19(4):201–4.
21. Dan M, Somer I, Knobel B, Gutman R. Cutaneous manifestations of infection with Corynebacterium group JK. Rev Infect Dis. 1988;10(6):1204–7.
22. Rezaei Bookani K, Marcus R, Cheikh E, Parish M, Salahuddin U. Corynebacterium jeikeium endocarditis: a case report and comprehensive review of an underestimated infection. IDCases. 2018;11:26–30.
23. Ramanan P, Barreto JN, Osmon DR, Tosh PK. Rothia bacteremia: a 10-year experience at Mayo Clinic, Rochester, Minnesota. J Clin Microbiol. 2014;52(9):3184–9.
24. Salminen MK, Rautelin H, Tynkkynen S, Poussa T, Saxelin M, Valtonen V, et al. Lactobacillus bacteremia, clinical significance, and patient outcome, with special focus on probiotic L. rhamnosus. GG Clin Infect Dis: Off Publ Infect Dis Soc Am. 2004;38(1):62–9.
25. Antony SJ. Lactobacillemia: an emerging cause of infection in both the immunocompromised and the immunocompetent host. J Natl Med Assoc. 2000;92(2):83–6.
26. Lassmann B, Gustafson DR, Wood CM, Rosenblatt JE. Reemergence of anaerobic bacteremia. Clin Infect Dis. 2007;44(7):895–900.
27. Noriega LM, Van der Auwera P, Phan M, Daneau D, Meunier F, Gerain J, et al. Anaerobic bacteremia in a cancer center. Support Care Cancer: Off J Multinat Assoc Support Care Cancer. 1993;1(5):250–5.
28. Zahar JR, Farhat H, Chachaty E, Meshaka P, Antoun S, Nitenberg G. Incidence and clinical significance of anaerobic bacteraemia in cancer patients: a 6-year retrospective study. Clin Microbiol Infect. 2005;11(9):724–9.
29. Riordan T. Human infection with Fusobacterium necrophorum (Necrobacillosis), with a focus on Lemierre's syndrome. Clin Microbiol Rev. 2007;20(4):622–59.
30. Centor RM, Atkinson TP, Ratliff AE, Xiao L, Crabb DM, Estrada CA, et al. The clinical presentation of Fusobacterium-positive and streptococcal-positive pharyngitis in a university health clinic: a cross-sectional study. Ann Intern Med. 2015;162(4):241–7.
31. Candoni A, Fili C, Trevisan R, Silvestri F, Fanin R. Fusobacterium nucleatum: a rare cause of bacteremia in neutropenic patients with leukemia and lymphoma. Clin Microbiol Infect. 2003;9(11):1112–5.
32. Landsaat PM, van der Lelie H, Bongaerts G, Kuijper EJ. Fusobacterium nucleatum, a new invasive pathogen in neutropenic patients? Scand J Infect Dis. 1995;27(1):83–4.
33. Jensen A, Hansen TM, Bank S, Kristensen LH, Prag J. Fusobacterium necrophorum tonsillitis: an important cause of tonsillitis in adolescents and young adults. Clin Microbiol Infect: Off Publ Eur Soc Clin Microbiol Infect Dis. 2015;21(3):266.e1–3.
34. Gustinetti G, Mikulska M. Bloodstream infections in neutropenic cancer patients: a practical update. Virulence. 2016;7(3):280–97.
35. Olson D, Yacoub AT, Gjini AD, Domingo G, Greene JN. Escherichia coli: an important pathogen in patients with hematologic malignancies. Mediterranean J Hematol Infect Dis. 2014;6(1):e2014068.
36. Carratala J, Fernandez-Sevilla A, Tubau F, Callis M, Gudiol F. Emergence of quinolone-resistant Escherichia coli bacteremia in neutropenic patients with cancer who have received prophylactic norfloxacin. Clin Infect Dis. 1995;20(3):557–60.. discussion 61–3
37. Krcmery V, Spanik S, Mrazova M, Trupl J, Grausova S, Grey E, et al. Bacteremias caused by Escherichia coli in cancer patients – analysis of 65 episodes. Int J Infect Dis: IJID: Off Publ Int Soc Infect Dis. 2002;6(1):69–73.
38. Ko WC, Paterson DL, Sagnimeni AJ, Hansen DS, Von Gottberg A, Mohapatra S, et al. Community-acquired Klebsiella pneumoniae bacteremia: global differences in clinical patterns. Emerg Infect Dis. 2002;8(2):160–6.

39. Tofas P, Skiada A, Angelopoulou M, Sipsas N, Pavlopoulou I, Tsaousi S, et al. Carbapenemase-producing Klebsiella pneumoniae bloodstream infections in neutropenic patients with haematological malignancies or aplastic anaemia: analysis of 50 cases. Int J Antimicrob Agents. 2016;47(4):335–9.
40. Girometti N, Lewis RE, Giannella M, Ambretti S, Bartoletti M, Tedeschi S, et al. Klebsiella pneumoniae bloodstream infection: epidemiology and impact of inappropriate empirical therapy. Medicine. 2014;93(17):298–309.
41. Kang CI, Kim SH, Kim HB, Park SW, Choe YJ, Oh MD, et al. Pseudomonas aeruginosa bacteremia: risk factors for mortality and influence of delayed receipt of effective antimicrobial therapy on clinical outcome. Clin Infect Dis. 2003;37(6):745–51.
42. Micek ST, Lloyd AE, Ritchie DJ, Reichley RM, Fraser VJ, Kollef MH. Pseudomonas aeruginosa bloodstream infection: importance of appropriate initial antimicrobial treatment. Antimicrob Agents Chemother. 2005;49(4):1306–11.
43. Kim HS, Park BK, Kim SK, Han SB, Lee JW, Lee DG, et al. Clinical characteristics and outcomes of Pseudomonas aeruginosa bacteremia in febrile neutropenic children and adolescents with the impact of antibiotic resistance: a retrospective study. BMC Infect Dis. 2017;17(1):500.
44. Kim YJ, Jun YH, Kim YR, Park KG, Park YJ, Kang JY, et al. Risk factors for mortality in patients with Pseudomonas aeruginosa bacteremia; retrospective study of impact of combination antimicrobial therapy. BMC Infect Dis. 2014;14:161.
45. Lopez-Calleja AI, Morilla Morales E, Nunez Medina R, Fernandez Esgueva M, Sahagun Pareja J, Garcia-Lechuz Moya JM, et al. Antimicrobial activity of ceftolozane-tazobactam against multidrug-resistant and extensively drug-resistant Pseudomonas aeruginosa clinical isolates from a Spanish hospital. Revista espanola de quimioterapia : publicacion oficial de la Sociedad Espanola de Quimioterapia. 2019;32(1):68–72.
46. Micozzi A, Venditti M, Monaco M, Friedrich A, Taglietti F, Santilli S, et al. Bacteremia due to Stenotrophomonas maltophilia in patients with hematologic malignancies. Clin Infect Dis. 2000;31(3):705–11.
47. Cho SY, Lee DG, Choi SM, Park C, Chun HS, Park YJ, et al. Stenotrophomonas maltophilia bloodstream infection in patients with hematologic malignancies: a retrospective study and in vitro activities of antimicrobial combinations. BMC Infect Dis. 2015;15:69.
48. Gokhan Gozel M, Celik C, Elaldi N. Stenotrophomonas maltophilia infections in adults: primary bacteremia and pneumonia. Jundishapur J Microbiol. 2015;8(8):e23569.
49. Al-Anazi KA, Al-Jasser AM. Infections caused by Stenotrophomonas maltophilia in recipients of hematopoietic stem cell transplantation. Front Oncol. 2014;4:232.
50. Wei C, Ni W, Cai X, Zhao J, Cui J. Evaluation of trimethoprim/sulfamethoxazole (SXT), minocycline, tigecycline, moxifloxacin, and ceftazidime alone and in combinations for SXT-susceptible and SXT-resistant stenotrophomonas maltophilia by in vitro time-kill experiments. PLoS One. 2016;11(3):e0152132.
51. Looney WJ, Narita M, Muhlemann K. Stenotrophomonas maltophilia: an emerging opportunist human pathogen. Lancet Infect Dis. 2009;9(5):312–23.
52. Ballo O, Tarazzit I, Stratmann J, Reinheimer C, Hogardt M, Wichelhaus TA, et al. Colonization with multidrug resistant organisms determines the clinical course of patients with acute myeloid leukemia undergoing intensive induction chemotherapy. PLoS One. 2019;14(1):e0210991.
53. Satlin MJ, Cohen N, Ma KC, Gedrimaite Z, Soave R, Askin G, et al. Bacteremia due to carbapenem-resistant Enterobacteriaceae in neutropenic patients with hematologic malignancies. J Inf Secur. 2016;73(4):336–45.
54. Yigit H, Queenan AM, Anderson GJ, Domenech-Sanchez A, Biddle JW, Steward CD, et al. Novel carbapenem-hydrolyzing beta-lactamase, KPC-1, from a carbapenem-resistant strain of Klebsiella pneumoniae. Antimicrob Agents Chemother. 2001;45(4):1151–61.
55. Yong D, Toleman MA, Giske CG, Cho HS, Sundman K, Lee K, et al. Characterization of a new metallo-beta-lactamase gene, bla(NDM-1), and a novel erythromycin esterase gene carried on a unique genetic structure in Klebsiella pneumoniae sequence type 14 from India. Antimicrob Agents Chemother. 2009;53(12):5046–54.

56. Turton JF, Ward ME, Woodford N, Kaufmann ME, Pike R, Livermore DM, et al. The role of ISAba1 in expression of OXA carbapenemase genes in Acinetobacter baumannii. FEMS Microbiol Lett. 2006;258(1):72–7.
57. Parruti G, Frattari A, Polilli E, Savini V, Sciacca A, Consorte A, et al. Cure of recurring Klebsiella pneumoniae carbapenemase-producing Klebsiella pneumoniae septic shock episodes due to complicated soft tissue infection using a ceftazidime and avibactam-based regimen: a case report. J Med Case Rep. 2019;13(1):20.
58. Athans V, Neuner EA, Hassouna H, Richter SS, Keller G, Castanheira M, et al. Meropenem-vaborbactam as salvage therapy for ceftazidime-avibactam-resistant klebsiella pneumoniae bacteremia and abscess in a liver transplant recipient. Antimicrob Agents Chemother. 2019;63(1):1–8.
59. Marshall S, Hujer AM, Rojas LJ, Papp-Wallace KM, Humphries RM, Spellberg B, et al. Can ceftazidime-avibactam and aztreonam overcome beta-lactam resistance conferred by metallo-beta-lactamases in enterobacteriaceae? Antimicrob Agents Chemother. 2017;61(4):1–9.
60. Karaiskos I, Galani I, Souli M, Giamarellou H. Novel beta-lactam-beta-lactamase inhibitor combinations: expectations for the treatment of carbapenem-resistant Gram-negative pathogens. Expert Opin Drug Metab Toxicol. 2019;15(2):133–49.

Fungal Infections

Ana Paula Velez, Jorge Lamarche, and John N. Greene

Abstract The incidence of fungal infection in neutropenic patients is increasing as a result of new advances of chemotherapy, stem cell transplantation with associated immunosuppressive therapies, use of broad spectrum antibiotics, and central venous devices. As this susceptible population is living longer, even uncommon and more resistant fungal organisms can develop despite prophylactic antifungals.

This chapter will focus on common fungal infections seen in neutropenic patients, particularly yeast and molds. Endemic mycoses are not common in this population and will not be discussed in this chapter.

Keywords Candida Species · Non Candida yeast infections · Molds · Aspergillus · Fusarium · Scedosporium · Zygomecetes · Mucor · Dermatiaceous fungi · Hyalohyphomycosis · Mucorales

Yeast

Yeast exist widely in nature, as a result, humans are constantly exposed to many yeast genera. Depending on the host immune system and virulence factors of the yeast, patients can develop an infection.

With the increase of the immunosuppressed population, we are seeing a variety of yeast infections including some rare yeast only sporadically encountered before.

A. P. Velez, MD, FACP (✉)
Associate Professor, University of South Florida, Tampa, FL, USA
e-mail: ana.velez@moffitt.org

J. Lamarche, MD
USF Morsani College of Medicine James Haley VA Hospital, James Haley VA Hospital, Tampa, FL, USA

J. N. Greene, MD, FACP
USF Morsani College of Medicine, Moffitt Cancer Center and Research Institute, Tampa, FL, USA

A. P. Velez et al. (eds.), *Infections in Neutropenic Cancer Patients*,
https://doi.org/10.1007/978-3-030-21859-1_7

Candida Species

Candida spp are the absolutely dominant cause of yeast infections in neutropenic patients. *Candida spp* are part of the normal flora and subsequently invasive infections may arise when mucosal breakdown or impaired immune function occurs. There are at least 15 different *Candida spp* that can cause infections in humans (Table 1). The most commonly encountered species are *C. albicans, C. glabrata, C. krusei, C. parapsilosis and C. tropicalis* and in addition rarer species *C. guilliermondii, C. lusitaniae, C. kefyr, and C. dubliniensis* [1] [2]. The widespread use of antifungal prophylaxis such as azoles and echinocandins have been associated with a shift from *C. albicans* infections to various non albicans *Candida spp* in cancer patients [3].

Multidrug resistant *C. auris* has been associated with healthcare setting outbreaks. Outbrakes have occured in Japan in 2009 followed by S. Korea, India and now in more than a dozen countries resulting in a potential global threat [4, 5].

Clincal Manifestations, Diagnosis and Treatment

The most benign type of infections caused by *Candida spp* are due to local overgrowth of yeast on mucous membranes. These types of infections are orpharyngeal, esophagitis (for more details, please refer to the head and neck infections chapter) and vulvovaginitis.

The symptoms of candida vulvovaginitis are dysuria, dyspareunia, vulvar pruritus, erythema, and white discharge classically described as curd-like. The diagnosis can be made clinically and can be supported by detecting budding yeast on wet mount or KOH preparation.

Similarly, balanitis can be present as erythema of the penis with white patches associated with burning pain and pruritus. Candida vulvovaginitis and balanitis can spread to the groin, buttocks and thighs causing yeast intertrigo. The treatment of

Table 1 Yeast

Candida species	Non candida yeast species
C. albicans	*Cryptococcus spp*
C. glabrata	*Trichorsporon spp*
C. krusei	*Saccharomyces spp*
C. parapsilosis	*Rhodotorula spp*
C. tropicalis	*Malassezia spp*
C. guillermondii	*Blastoschyzomyces spp*
C. lusitaniae	
C. kefyr	
C. dubliniensis	
C. auris	

vulvovaginitis, balanitis and yeast intertrigo is with oral fluconazole or topical azoles such as clotrimazole, butoconazole, and miconazole [6]. For yeast intertrigo, topical nystatin can also be used [7].

Neutropenic patients are also at high risk for systemic candida infections leading to fungemia with visceral dissemination. The clinical manifestations are similar to bacteremia including fever (which may be absent), tachycardia and later hypotension complicated by multiorgan failure. Occasionally, erythematous painless macular, papular or pustular skin lesions on an erythematous base may be seen. These lesions may become necrotic. Biopsy of the skin lesions can be sent for KOH stain, culture and histopathology in order to facilitate the diagnosis.

Hepatosplenic candidiasis is a rare form of systemic candida infection seen almost exclusively in patients with hematologic malignancies who have recovered from neutropenia. Some patients had a documented episode of candidemia, but in other patients, the organism can spread from the portal circulation to the spleen and liver in the absence of clearly documented positive blood cultures. The clinical manifestations include fever and right upper quadrant pain in a patient who just recovered from neutropenia. Laboratory data reveals elevated serum alkaline phosphatase. The diagnosis can be suspected by visualizing multiple small hypo densities in the liver, spleen and kidney on computed tomography (CT), ultrasound, or magnetic resonance.

The treatment of uncomplicated candidemia without metastatic dissemination includes an echinocandin such as caspofungin, anidulafungin or micafungin until susceptibilities are available. Lipid formulation amphotericin B is another option, but less attractive given the potential nephrotoxicity. Voriconazole can be used when additional mold coverage is desired [1]. In patients who are already receiving an azole, an echinocandin or lipid formulation of amphotericin B can be added to treat potential *Candida spp* resistant to azole [1]. For patients who are already taking an echinocandin, voriconazole or lipid amphotericin B can be added to cover potential echinocandin resistant *Candida spp* [1]. The recommended duration of candidemia without a metastatic complication is 2 weeks after documented clearance of *Candida spp* from the bloodstream and provided that neutropenia has resolved [1]. Ophthalmology evaluation with dilated funduscopic examination should be performed within the first week of neutropenia resolution [1].

Treatment of the source of candidemia is of utmost importance to facilitate clearance and prevent relapse. In the neutropenic patient, the source of infection is usually translocation from the gastrointestinal tract. The decision of central line removal should be considered on an individual basis [1].

The initial treatment of hepatosplenic candidiasis includes lipid amphotericin B or an echinocandin for several weeks followed by oral fluconazole depending on the susceptibility of the yeast. Therapy should continue until the lesions resolve on repeated radiologic imaging. If additional chemotherapy or hematopoietic stem cell transplant is required, antifungal therapy should continue to prevent relapse of infection [1].

More specific information about the antifungal options and doses to use for the different species of candida is present in the chapter on Antifungal Medications in Neutropenia.

Non Candida Yeast Species

Non candida yeast infections in patients with neutropenia have the potential for lethal dissemination to distant organs, especially since they have natural resistance to many antifungal medications. There are many non-candida yeast sepecies that can cause infection in humans (Table 1). The most common organisms include *Cryptococcus spp*, *Trichosporon spp*, *Saccharomyces spp*, *Rhodotorula spp*, *Malassezia spp*, *Blastoschyzomyces spp*, and *Sporobolomyces spp*.

A retrospective analysis done in our institution found nine cases of non-candida yeast infections from 1999–2014. *Trichosporum beigelli* was the most common organism followed by *Blastoschizomyces capitatum* (previously known as *Trichosporum capitatun*, later as *Geotrichum capitatum*) and lastly *Sporothrix cyanescens* [8].

Clincal Manifestations and Treatment

For the most part, non-candida yeast infections encountered in neutropenic patients cause similar symptomatology and spectrum of disease. Invasive and systemic disease is very similar to systemic candidiasis and hepatosplenic candidiasis. These organisms can invade any organ in the human body [9–14]. This is particularly true for *Trischosporion spp.* which can also cause diffuse alveolar hemorrhage [15, 16].

Diagnosis is suspected when a patient with prolonged neutropenia has fever, with or without skin lesions and imaging testing reveals small hepatic or splenic lesions. Erythematous macular or papular lesions similar to those seen in disseminated candida infection can also be seen. The diagnosis lies in isolating the organism in blood, urine, sputum or spinal fluid [9, 15, 17]. If skin lesions are present, culture and histopathology can also isolate the fungus. To isolate *Malassezia spp* in blood culture, a lipid enriched media is required [12].

Treatment should be individualized for each species. Given the unpredictable activity of antifungals against these organisms, in vitro susceptibilities should be done on all isolates and antifungals should be tailored pending the susceptibility of the testing [9, 13].

In general most *Trichosporon spp* have a high minimal inhibitory concentration (MIC's) for polyenes, flucytosine, and echinocandins, with relatively low MICs for the azoles. Among the azoles, voriconazole and posaconazole appear to be the best option

[18]. Combination therapy may be tried in patients failing azole treatment. Combination includes an azole with an echinocandin or amphotericin B with micafungin [19].

Rhodotorula spp have in vitro susceptibility to amphotericin B and fluocytosine, but are resistant to echinocandins and fluconazole. The newer triazoles have some activity, but more clinical experience is needed. Ravuconazole has excellent in vitro activity and may have a role in the future for life threatening infections [20].

The treatment of*Malassezia spp* includes prompt central catheter removal ideally with discontinuation of intravenous lipids if possible. In most cases, removal of the catheter may be sufficient for cure provided that there is no evidence of deep-seated infection [11]. In the setting of persistent fungemia or evidence of disseminated infection, systemic therapy is indicated. *Malassezia spp* are susceptible to azoles and polyenes, but are intrinsically resistant to flucytosine [9, 11].

Blastoschizomyces spp have in vitro susceptibility to amphotericin B, voriconazole and posaconazole. They are less susceptible to fluconazole and resistant to flucytosine and echinocandins [21, 22].

For infections secondary to *Saccharomyces spp central* line removal along with amphotericin B or fluconazole appears to be a good treatment option. Voriconazole may be used in patients failing fluconazole. Preliminary research and some case reports revealed that echinocandins may also be a good alternative for *Saccharomyces spp* [23, 24].

Given the morbidity and mortality of yeast non candida infections in neutropenic patients and their potential for dissemination, our initial approach when non candida yeast are isolated from the blood is to use double antifungal therapy with a lipid formulation of amphotericin B, and voriconazole until further identification and susceptibilities are available. Once more information is obtained, the antifungal therapy is tailored to the best option available.

Molds

Molds are common saprophytes in the environment. In immunosuppressed patients mold infections can be life threatening with several treatment challenges, especially if the underlying malignancy is not under control. Immunosuppressed patients may acquire an invasive mold infection by inhalation, blood stream infection from central catheters, or direct traumatic inoculation. Depending of the pathogen and host factors, the infection can spread locally to deeper tissues by angioinvasion or cause distant metastatic disease through conidia formation. In severe cases, a mold infection may have both, severe local angioinvasion with tissue necrosis plus distant metastatic invasion to vital organs. Molds can have septate or aseptate hyphae. They can also be pigmented or colorless (Table 2). This section will discussed some of the molds more commonly found in neutropenic patients.

Table 2 Mold

Hyalohyphomycosis Or hyaline molds Colorless septate hyphae	Zygomycetes -Mucorales Non septate hyphae	Phaeohyphomycosis Or dark molds Pigmented septate hyphae
Apergillus spp	*Rhizopus spp*	*Alternaria spp*
Fusarium spp	*Mucor spp*	*Exoophiala spp*
Scedosporium apiospermum	*Cunninghamella spp*	*Cladophialophora spp*
Penicillum spp	*Apophysomyces spp*	*Curvularia spp*
Paecilomyces spp	*Lichthenia spp*	*Phialemonium spp*
Acremonium spp	*Saksenaea spp*	*Exserohilum spp*
Scopulariopsis spp	*Rhizomucor spp*	*Microascus spp*
Beauveria spp		*Bipolaris spp*
		Ochroconis spp
		Chaetomium spp
		Cladosporium spp
		Phaeoacremonium spp
		Rhinocladiella spp

Hyalohyphomycosis

Hyalohyphomycosis is the term used to describe infections due to hyaline fungi. Hyaline fungi are colorless with septate hyphae under the microscope (Fig. 1). The most common hyaline fungi seen in neutropenic patients include *Aspergillus, Fusarium, Scedosporium apiospermum, Penicillium, Paecilomyces, Acremonium, Scopulariopsis,* and *Beauveria* (Table 2). *Lomentospora prolificans (*formerly *Scedosporium prolificans and* previously *Scedosporium inflatum)* are discussed in this section for clinical and practical purposes *but* they are phaeohyphomycosis or dark molds.

Among the organisms above, Aspergillus, Fusarium and Scedosporium are increasingly found in neutropenic patients therefore; this section will focus on these fungi.

Aspergillus

Among the *Aspergillus* spp, *A. fumigatus* is the most prevalent followed by *A. flavus, A. niger* and *A. terreus* [25].

Aspergillus is responsible for a number of clinical syndromes including allergic bronchopulmonary aspergillosis, and invasive pulmonary infections including chronic necrotizing pneumonia, invasive pulmonary aspergillosis, and sinusitis. In neutropenic patients the latter two forms are the most prevalent form of aspergillosis [26]. This could be explained partially by the inhalation of conidia which is the most common form of acquiring the infection. Occasionally traumatic inoculation and rarely gastrointestinal infection occur in neutropenic patients. Central nervous

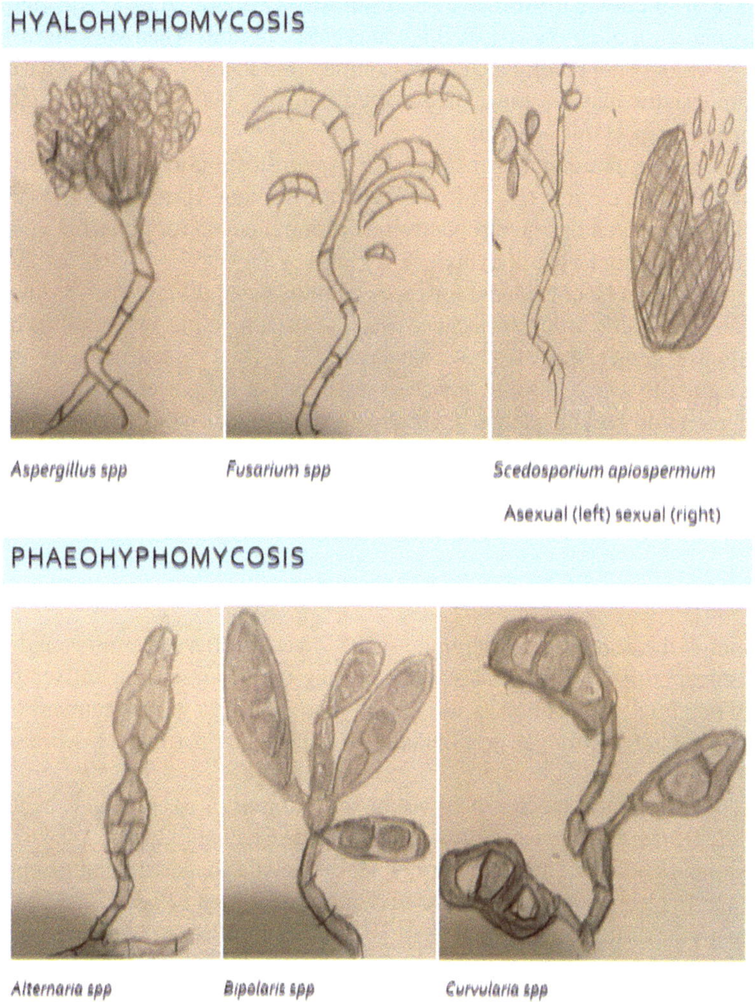

Fig. 1 (**a**) Hyalohyphomycosis. (**b**) Phaeohyphomycosis

system (CNS) dissemination is a life threatening consequence of disseminated aspergillosis. It can present as a new onset of seizures or even a stroke from a mass effect or angioinvasion of the CNS circulation [27].

The clinical manifestation, diagnosis and radiological findings of Aspergillus sinusitis and pneumonia are discussed in detail in this book under the chapter of Respiratory Infections in Neutropenia.

Triazoles are the preferred agent for treatment and prevention of invasive aspergillosis. Aerosolized amphotericin B can be an alternative for prophylaxis in neutropenic patients in whom the use of azoles is contraindicated [28]. Please refer to the chapter of Prophylaxis in Neutropenic Patients for more clear indications of Aspergillus prophylaxis.

The drug of choice for invasive Aspergillosis is voriconazole. Isavuconazole or lipid formulation of amphotericin B are alternative options when voriconazole cannot be given or is not readily available. Combination therapy with voriconazole and an echinocandin may be given in selected patients, but there is only moderate evidence to support this aproach.

The duration of treatment for invasive aspergillosis is 6–12 weeks or longer depending on the clinical and radiological improvement. If the patient is still neutropenic or if impending neutropenia is still anticipated, voriconazole should be continued for secondary prophylaxis [28].

Surgery should be considered for cases with localized disease such as cutaneous infection or sinusitis. In other instances such as osteomyelitis, endocarditis or focal CNS disease, surgery can also be considered [28].

For refractory cases, the emergence of resistance or the presence of an additional pathogen should be considered. Intensifying the regimen with another antifungal from a different class may be prudent in addition to tapering immunosuppressive therapy if possible [28].

Fusarium

Fusarium is the second most common mold infection after aspergillus and jointly with scedosporium and mucorales are increasing in the immunosuppressed population. A potential explanation is the newer immunosuppressive treatment and the extensive use of antifungal prophylaxis for aspergillus particularly voriconazole [29–31].

The most common species of fusarium are *F. solani, F. oxyosporum,* and *F. verticillioides (previously F. moniliforme) and F. proliferatum* [32, 33].

The macroconidia of fusarium are typically banana shaped and multiseptate. In tissue, the hyphae are septate similar to *Aspergilus spp* and *Pseudaslleschería spp* making it very difficult to distinguish these fungi in the absence of microbial growth [32, 34]. However, fusarium is more likely to have balloing hyphae.

Fusarium is ubiquitous in water and soil and can cause superficial and subcutaneous infection with local deep angioinvasion with distant spread particularly in immunosuppressed patients [33, 35]. Immunosuppressed patients acquire the infection by inhalation of spores, or direct inoculation. The latter can be seen in neutropenic patients with toe nail trauma. The nail and the periungual area can be colonized with fusarium spores that can invade locally after toe-nail trauma. Subsequently the infection can spread via the lymphatic and blood vassels to reach vital organs causing life threatening infection [36]. Because of its ability to spread distantly, the mold can be occasionally isolated in blood cultures. This is a very unique characteristic of fusarium in contrast to other molds [33, 37].

The clinical manifestation of fusarium infections differ in immunocompetent versus immunosuppressed patients. Superficial or localized infections can be seen in immunocompetent patients whereas complicated deeper infection involving the sinuses, lungs and the more common disseminated disease can be seen in immunosuppressed patients [33, 38]. The clinical manifestations of sinusitis and pneumonia caused by fusarium resembles aspergillus infection, but contrary to aspergillus, fusarium is more likely to cause skin lesions from traumatic inoculation, onychomycosis with periungual toe infection and secondary systemic infection [36, 39].

Localized skin infections initially present with severe painful erythema at the site of inoculation. Often it is the periungual area, but can present anywhere in the body. The lesions later progress to develop a purpuric center that later becomes necrotic resembling ecthyma gangrenosum. Secondary lymphangitic spread with or without secondary metastatic skin lesions can also be seen. These secondary skin lesions are also painful and can progress from small papular erythematous lesions to large nodules with central necrosis. Some of them can also have the appearance of target lesions.

The definitive diagnosis of disseminated fusarium is by isolating the organism in culture from blood, skin, tissue, sputum or by histopathology of the affected tissue. Molecular diagnosis is often required for more specific detail about the species [33, 40].

The treatment of fusarium infections represents a challenge. Some of the species are intrinsically resistant to several antifungals. Liposomal formulation of amphotericin B and voriconazole are the most active antifungals and can be used in combination therapy until more information regarding susceptibility results are available [33, 41–44]. Other combination therapies that can be synergistic include voriconazole plus terbinafine [33, 45]. Posaconazole has also been used as salvage therapy [46]. Isavuconazole is a new azole approved for the treatment of mucormycosis and aspergillosis but clinical experience for treatment of fusarium infections is limited. Antifungal susceptibility testing allows for more specific treatment and should be done to improve the patient's outcome. Removal of the infected catheter if thought to be the source of infection, should be done. If the primary source of infection is the toe nail, removal is necessary as it can serve as a nidus of persistent infection [36]. Immunomodulation with G-CSF or GM-CSF plus interferon gamma can be used as an adjunctive therapy in addition to antifungals [41].

The duration of treatment is usually prolonged for several weeks until there is clinical and radiological evidence of improvement. Treatment should also continue until resolution of neutropenia. If chemotherapy or neutropenia is anticipated, secondary prophylaxis should be given during the periods of increased immunosuppression such as treatment of graft vs. host disease [38].

In general fusarium infection in immunosuppressed patients is lethal in spite of aggressive antifungal treatment. The overall prognosis largely depends on the degree of immunosuppression and the extent of infection. Recovery of neutropenia is an essential factor for survival [39, 47].

Scedosporium

There are two species of Scedosporium that can cause disease in humans, *S. apiospermum,* its sexual form *Pseudallescheria boydii and Lomentospora prolificans* (formerly *Scedosporium prolificans* and previously *Scedosporium inflatum*) [41, 48–50] Scedosporium has been isolated widely in the environment including soil, potting mix, compost and polluted water. Infection occurs by direct inoculation or inhalation of conidia.

In the immunocompetent host the spectrum of disease includes keratitis, endopthalmitis, cutaneous and subcutaneous infection (Mycetoma), and osteomyelitis. Given the neurotropic nature of this mold, meningoencephalitis, brain abscess, in addition to sinusitis and pneumonia have also been described in near drowning accidents [33, 41, 49].

In immunocompromised patients, the clinical manifestations is very similar to fusarium infections including sinusitis, pneumonia, and disseminated disease with skin lesions similar to the ones described previously for fusarium. In addition, CNS infections including meningitis, meningoencephalitis and brain abscess can also occur. Disseminated infection is more commonly reported with *L. prolificans* than *S. apiospermum* [51]. Similarly to fusarium infections, blood cultures can be positive for mold. Local infection can also metastasize to distant organs [49, 52].

The diagnosis of Scedosporium relies on isolation of the organisms on histopathology or cultures from tissue, sputum or blood. Invasive pulmonary infections, sinusitis or CNS infections are indistinguishable radiologically from aspergillus or fusarium [33, 49]. Molecular testing allows for more specific information regarding the species but unfortunately is not available in most centers [41].

The optimal choice and duration of treatment for Scedosporium infections is unknown. Infections caused by these organisms in immunosuppressed patients are often disseminated and carry mortality rates from 40 to 100% [49, 51].

Among the antifungals, voriconazole appears to be the best option. MICs from *S. apiospermum* for voriconazole are better than the MICs for *L. prolificans* [53]. Isavuconazole is not approved for the treatment of scedosporium but in vitro data shows that it may have activity [41]. Ampothericin B is not active in general for scedosporium infections and echinocandins have decreased susceptibilities. Given the high rates of resistance, susceptibility testing is highly recommended [41, 54].

Because of the aggressive nature of scedosporium especially *L. prolificans* and the relative high MIC to voriconazole, some experts advocate combination therapy with voriconazole plus a polyene or an echinocandin [41]. Triple antifungal therapy with voriconazole, an echinocandin and a polyene has been tested against *L. prolificans* showing in vitro synergy but the data in humans is limited [41]. Clinical experience with the use of immunomodulation therapy with G-CSF or GM-CSF combined with interferon gamma is limited [33, 41].

Zygomycetes

Zygomecetes are distributed worldwide in the soil and decaying vegetation. They have gained recent popularity because of the increase in the number of cases in the immunosuppressed population particularly in the last decade [55]. This could be partly because of the widespread use of voriconazole as prophylaxis or treatment of aspergillosis [31, 56].

Zygomyecetes are characterized in culture by broad nonseptate ribbonlike hyphae. There are two main groups of zygomecetes; entomophthorales and mucorales. The entomophthorales mainly cause cutaneous and subcutaneous infections and is limited to the tropics. The mucorales group can cause severe and lethal angioinvasive infections involving the respiratory, gastrointestinal, genitourinary and cutaneous systems. Most of these infections are severe because they can invade the blood vessels causing thrombosis with secondary tissue necrosis [55–58].

The most common organisms that belong to mucorales is *Rhizopus* followed by *Mucor*. Other less common organisms from the genus of mucorales include *Cunninghamella, Apophysomyces, Lichtheimia* (formerly *Absidia*), *Saksenaea*, and *Rhizomucor* [59].

Predisposing factors for infection include diabetes, steroid use, deferoxamine therapy, iron overload, trauma, hematological malignancies and transplant recipients, specially while taking voriconazole prophylaxis [60–63].

The infection is acquired by inhalation of spores or direct inoculation. The most common clinical form of presentation is rhino-orbital-cerebral. This clinical presentation is more commonly seen in diabetic and other immunosuppressed patients. The clinical symptoms include fever, sinus congestion, pain, and headache. This infection can cause angioinvasion and spread to nearby tissues including the palate and brain. On physical examination, a palate or nose eschar can be present. In addition, peri-orbital erythema, edema and proptosis can be seen [64].

In patients with hematological malignancy, the most common site of infection is the lung [55]. The clinical symptoms of pneumonia do not differ from other mold infections in the immunosuppressed patient. Patients may present with fever, cough and pleuritic pain or may be asymptomatic. A new large lung nodule with or without the reverse halo sign may be discovered incidentally on CT scan.

Cutaneous infection caused by zygomycosis also does not differ from any other mold infection in immunosuppressed patients. The initial presentation may be a painful papular or plaque lesion at the site of inoculation. This lesion rapidly enlarges and develops surrounding erythema with a necrotic center [65]. This lesion rapidly spreads to deeper tissues causing necrosis with unfavorable consequences.

The diagnosis of zygomycetes relies on isolation of the organism from histopathology and culture from tissues or sputum. Molecular studies are not readily available in most institutions. Efforts to obtain biopsies particularly from the sinuses and the skin should be pursued. Unfortunately, thrombocytopenia is usually present in neutropenic patients; therefore, biopsy is not always possible especially from the lung because of the unacceptable high risk of bleeding.

Radiological findings of lung infection may reveal the reverse halo sign (please refer to the chapter of Pulmonary Infections in Neutropenia for more details). Sputum samples should be obtained, and if negative, broncholaveolar lavage should be obtained. In cases of suspected mold sinusitis, ears, nose, and throat endoscopic examination should be done and repeated for follow up of treatment response. In addition, tissue samples should be obtained for histopathology and culture [55, 66].

The treatment of zygomycosis includes surgical debridement if there is evidence of skin, soft tissue infection or rhinocerebral infection, in addition to antifungal therapy. Amphotericin B, posaconazole and isavuconazole are all active in vitro [55, 66].

The first line of therapy is lipid formulation of amphotericin B. Posaconazole also has activity but is only indicated as alternative therapy [55, 67]. In a multicenter open –label single arm study isavuconazole showed showed similar efficacy to amphotericin B, but isavuconazole has not been studied in randomized trials [68]. Posaconazole and isavuconazole can be used for step down therapy after the patient has shown signs of improvement with amphotericin B.

Data for combination therapy with lipid formulation of amphotericin B with either an echinocandin or posaconazole is insufficient and controversial [55, 69, 70]. Combination therapy should be a bedside decision outweighing risk vs. benefits. Efforts to treat the malignancy and decrease the immunosuppression should be a priority [69, 70].

The length of treatment is usually from several weeks to months until there is clinical and radiological evidence of resolution. Maintenance therapy or secondary prophylaxis should be considered if persistent immunosuppression continues [55].

Similar to other invasive mold infections, the prognosis for zygomyces infection largely depends on resolution of neutropenia and immunosuppression. Antifungals alone in the presence of ongoing immunosuppression will not ensure cure.

Phaeohyphomycosis

Dematiaceous fungi are darkly pigmented due to melanin-like pigments in the cell wall. These pigments cause the hyphae to have the appearance of a golden brown color under the microscope. The hyphae are septate just like the hyphae of hyaline molds (Fig. 1). Dermatiaceous fungi rarely cause disease in humans but are increasingly seen in immunocompromised patients.

The dematiaceous fungi are found in the soil and decaying vegetation of tropical and subtropical areas. The most common organisms associated with phaeohyphomicosis in immunosuppressed patients include *Alternaria, Exophiala, Cladophialophora, Curvularia, Phialemonium, Exserohilum, Microascus, Bipolaris, Ochroconis, Chaetomium, Cladosporium, Phaeoacremonium,* and *Rhinocladiella* [71, 72] (Table 2).

Lomentospora prolificans (formerly *Scedosporium prolificans* and previously *Scedosporium inflatum*) is also part of the phaeohyphomycosis which was described under the hyalohyphomycosis for clinical and practical purposes.

It is important to highlight that these molds have neurotrophic characteristics that frequently lead to CNS infections. The rest of the clinical syndromes are similar to other molds described previously in this chapter including cutaneous and subcutaneous infections, pneumonia, fungemia and disseminated disease [71, 72].

The diagnosis is by histopathology and microscopic examination of cultures. Microscopic examination yields fungal elements with dark cell walls with branching septate hyphae that usually look brown in most stains. Occasionally the Fontana-Masson stain specific for melanin can be used [73].

The treatment for cutaneous and CNS infections is surgical debridement in addition to antifungals [71]. Unfortunately the resistance patterns are highly variable among phaeohyphomycosis and there are no clear guidelines for treatment. Antifungals often used to treat these infections include voriconazole, posaconazole and amphotericin B [72]. Combination therapy has also been used with triazoles, amphotericin B, and an echinocandin [72]. Treatment is often continued for several months until clinical symptoms and the immunosuppression resolve [71, 72].

References

1. Pappas PG, Kauffman CA, Andes DR, Clancy CJ, Marr KA, Ostrosky-Zeichner L, et al. Clinical practice guideline for the management of candidiasis: 2016 update by the Infectious Diseases Society of America. Clin Infect Dis. 2016;62(4):e1–50.
2. Arendrup MC. Candida and candidaemia. Susceptibility and epidemiology. Dan Med J. 2013;60(11):B4698.
3. Jung DS, Farmakiotis D, Jiang Y, Tarrand JJ, Kontoyiannis DP. Uncommon Candida species Fungemia among cancer patients, Houston, Texas, USA. Emerg Infect Dis. 2015;21(11):1942–50.
4. Tsay S, Kallen A, Jackson BR, Chiller TM, Vallabhaneni S. Approach to the investigation and management of patients with Candida auris, an emerging multidrug-resistant yeast. Clin Infect Dis. 2018;66(2):306–11.
5. Saris K, Meis JF, Voss A. Candida auris. Curr Opin Infect Dis. 2018;31(4):34–340.
6. Dovnik A, Golle A, Novak D, Arko D, Takac I. Treatment of vulvovaginal candidiasis: a review of the literature. Acta dermatovenerologica Alpina, Pannonica, et Adriatica. 2015;24(1):5–7.
7. Metin A, Dilek N, Bilgili SG. Recurrent candidal intertrigo: challenges and solutions. Clin Cosmet Investig Dermatol. 2018;11:175–85.
8. Prodhan T, Yacoub AT, Jones L, Mai J, Greene J. Non-candida yeasts fungemia in cancer patients: a retrospective analysis at a referral cancer center, 1999–2014. Infect Dis Clin Pract. 2015;23(5):260–2.
9. Hazen KC. New and emerging yeast pathogens. Clin Microbiol Rev. 1995;8(4):462–78.
10. Marcon MJ, Powell DA. Epidemiology, diagnosis, and management of Malassezia furfur systemic infection. Diagn Microbiol Infect Dis. 1987;7(3):161–75.
11. Marcon MJ, Powell DA. Human infections due to Malassezia spp. Clin Microbiol Rev. 1992;5(2):101–19.
12. Iatta R, Cafarchia C, Cuna T, Montagna O, Laforgia N, Gentile O, et al. Bloodstream infections by Malassezia and Candida species in critical care patients. Med Mycol. 2014;52(3):264–9.

13. Martino P, Venditti M, Micozzi A, Morace G, Polonelli L, Mantovani MP, et al. Blastoschizomyces capitatus: an emerging cause of invasive fungal disease in leukemia patients. Rev Infect Dis. 1990;12(4):570–82.
14. Tsiodras S, Papageorgiou S, Meletiadis J, Tofas P, Pappa V, Panayiotides J, et al. Rhodotorula mucilaginosa associacted meningitis: a subacute entity with high mortality. Case report and review. Med Mycol Case Rep. 2014;6:46–50.
15. Tashiro T, Nagai H, Nagaoka H, Goto Y, Kamberi P, Nasu M. Trichosporon beigelii pneumonia in patients with hematologic malignancies. Chest. 1995;108(1):190–5.
16. Ebright JR, Fairfax MR, Vazquez JA. Trichosporon asahii, a non-candida yeast that caused fatal septic shock in a patient without cancer or neutropenia. Clin Infect Dis. 2001;33(5):E28–30.
17. Surmont I, Vergauwen B, Marcelis L, Verbist L, Verhoef G, Boogaerts M. First report of chronic meningitis caused by Trichosporon beigelii. European journal of clinical microbiology & infectious diseases : official publication of the. Eur Soc Clin Microbiol. 1990;9(3):226–9.
18. Paphitou NI, Ostrosky-Zeichner L, Paetznick VL, Rodriguez JR, Chen E, Rex JH. In vitro antifungal susceptibilities of Trichosporon species. Antimicrob Agents Chemother. 2002;46(4):1144–6.
19. Serena C, Pastor FJ, Gilgado F, Mayayo E, Guarro J. Efficacy of micafungin in combination with other drugs in a murine model of disseminated trichosporonosis. Antimicrob Agents Chemother. 2005;49(2):497–502.
20. Diekema DJ, Petroelje B, Messer SA, Hollis RJ, Pfaller MA. Activities of available and investigational antifungal agents against rhodotorula species. J Clin Microbiol. 2005;43(1):476–8.
21. Koc AN, Copur Cicek A, Kaynar L, Sav H, Kasap Tekinsen FF, Atalay MA. Three cases of fungemia caused by Blastoschizomyces capitatus. Mikrobiyoloji bulteni. 2013;47(4):734–41.
22. Espinel-Ingroff A. Comparison of in vitro activities of the new triazole SCH56592 and the echinocandins MK-0991 (L-743,872) and LY303366 against opportunistic filamentous and dimorphic fungi and yeasts. J Clin Microbiol. 1998;36(10):2950–6.
23. Enache-Angoulvant A, Hennequin C. Invasive Saccharomyces infection: a comprehensive review. Clin Infect Dis. 2005;41(11):1559–68.
24. Popiel KY, Wong P, Lee MJ, Langelier M, Sheppard DC, Vinh DC. Invasive Saccharomyces cerevisiae in a liver transplant patient: case report and review of infection in transplant recipients. Transpl Infect Dis: Off J Transpl Soc. 2015;17(3):435–41.
25. Marr KA, Carter RA, Crippa F, Wald A, Corey L. Epidemiology and outcome of mould infections in hematopoietic stem cell transplant recipients. Clin Infect Dis. 2002;34(7):909–17.
26. Abers MS, Ghebremichael MS, Timmons AK, Warren HS, Poznansky MC, Vyas JM. A critical reappraisal of prolonged neutropenia as a risk factor for invasive pulmonary aspergillosis. Open Forum Infect Dis. 2016;3(1):ofw036.
27. Segal BH. Aspergillosis. N Engl J Med. 2009;360(18):1870–84.
28. Patterson TF, Thompson GR 3rd, Denning DW, Fishman JA, Hadley S, Herbrecht R, et al. Executive summary: practice guidelines for the diagnosis and management of aspergillosis: 2016 update by the Infectious Diseases Society of America. Clin Infect Dis. 2016;63(4):433–42.
29. Peman J, Salavert M. Invasive fungal disease due to Scedosporium, Fusarium and mucorales. Revista iberoamericana de micologia. 2014;31(4):242–8.
30. Walsh TJ, Gamaletsou MN. Treatment of fungal disease in the setting of neutropenia. Hematology Am Soc Hematol Educ Program. 2013;2013:423–7.
31. Lamoth F, Chung SJ, Damonti L, Alexander BD. Changing epidemiology of invasive mold infections in patients receiving azole prophylaxis. Clin Infect Dis. 2017;64(11):1619–21.
32. Nelson PE, Dignani MC, Anaissie EJ. Taxonomy, biology, and clinical aspects of Fusarium species. Clin Microbiol Rev. 1994;7(4):479–504.
33. Tortorano AM, Richardson M, Roilides E, van Diepeningen A, Caira M, Munoz P, et al. ESCMID and ECMM joint guidelines on diagnosis and management of hyalohyphomycosis: Fusarium spp., Scedosporium spp. and others. Clinical microbiology and infection : the official publication of the European Society of Clinical. Microbiol Infect Dis. 2014;20 (Suppl 3):27–46.

34. Hayden RT, Isotalo PA, Parrett T, Wolk DM, Qian X, Roberts GD, et al. In situ hybridization for the differentiation of Aspergillus, Fusarium, and Pseudallescheria species in tissue section. Diagn Molecul Pathol: Am J Surg Pathol, Part B. 2003;12(1):21–6.
35. Boutati EI, Anaissie EJ. Fusarium, a significant emerging pathogen in patients with hematologic malignancy: ten years' experience at a cancer center and implications for management. Blood. 1997;90(3):999–1008.
36. Velez A, Greene J, L. Vincent A, M. Elko-Simms Impact and etiology of periungual toe infections in neutropenic patients. Infectious Diseases in Clinical Practice. 2012;20(6):e31–e34.
37. Liu K, Howell DN, Perfect JR, Schell WA. Morphologic criteria for the preliminary identification of Fusarium, Paecilomyces, and Acremonium species by histopathology. Am J Clin Pathol. 1998;109(1):45–54.
38. Nucci M, Anaissie E. Fusarium infections in immunocompromised patients. Clin Microbiol Rev. 2007;20(4):695–704.
39. Nucci F, Nouer SA, Capone D, Anaissie E, Nucci M. Fusariosis. Semin Respir Crit Care Med. 2015;36(5):706–14.
40. Hue FX, Huerre M, Rouffault MA, de Bievre C. Specific detection of fusarium species in blood and tissues by a PCR technique. J Clin Microbiol. 1999;37(8):2434–8.
41. McCarthy MW, Katragkou A, Iosifidis E, Roilides E, Walsh TJ. Recent advances in the treatment of scedosporiosis and fusariosis. J Fungi (Basel, Switzerland). 2018;4(2):1–16.
42. Tupaki-Sreepurna A, Kindo AJ. Fusarium: the versatile pathogen. Indian J Med Microbiol. 2018;36(1):8–17.
43. Taj-Aldeen SJ. Reduced multidrug susceptibility profile is a common feature of opportunistic fusarium species: fusarium multi-drug resistant pattern. J Fungi (Basel, Switzerland). 2017;3(2):1–15.
44. Al-Hatmi AMS, Bonifaz A, Ranque S, Sybren de Hoog G, Verweij PE, Meis JF. Current antifungal treatment of fusariosis. Int J Antimicrob Agents. 2018;51(3):326–32.
45. Cordoba S, Rodero L, Vivot W, Abrantes R, Davel G, Vitale RG. In vitro interactions of antifungal agents against clinical isolates of Fusarium spp. Int J Antimicrob Agents. 2008;31(2):171–4.
46. Raad II, Hachem RY, Herbrecht R, Graybill JR, Hare R, Corcoran G, et al. Posaconazole as salvage treatment for invasive fusariosis in patients with underlying hematologic malignancy and other conditions. Clin Infect Dis. 2006;42(10):1398–403.
47. Nucci M, Anaissie E. Emerging fungi. Infect Dis Clin N Am. 2006;20(3):563–79.
48. Gilgado F, Cano J, Gene J, Guarro J. Molecular phylogeny of the Pseudallescheria boydii species complex: proposal of two new species. J Clin Microbiol. 2005;43(10):4930–42.
49. Cortez KJ, Roilides E, Quiroz-Telles F, Meletiadis J, Antachopoulos C, Knudsen T, et al. Infections caused by Scedosporium spp. Clin Microbiol Rev. 2008;21(1):157–97.
50. Ramirez-Garcia A, Pellon A, Rementeria A, Buldain I, Barreto-Bergter E, Rollin-Pinheiro R, et al. Scedosporium and Lomentospora: an updated overview of underrated opportunists. Med Mycol. 2018;56(suppl_1):102–25.
51. Husain S, Munoz P, Forrest G, Alexander BD, Somani J, Brennan K, et al. Infections due to Scedosporium apiospermum and Scedosporium prolificans in transplant recipients: clinical characteristics and impact of antifungal agent therapy on outcome. Clin Infect Dis. 2005;40(1):89–99.
52. Berenguer J, Rodriguez-Tudela JL, Richard C, Alvarez M, Sanz MA, Gaztelurrutia L, et al. Deep infections caused by Scedosporium prolificans. A report on 16 cases in Spain and a review of the literature. Scedosporium Prolificans Spanish Study Group Medicine. 1997;76(4):256–65.
53. Troke P, Aguirrebengoa K, Arteaga C, Ellis D, Heath CH, Lutsar I, et al. Treatment of scedosporiosis with voriconazole: clinical experience with 107 patients. Antimicrob Agents Chemother. 2008;52(5):1743–50.
54. Gilgado F, Serena C, Cano J, Gene J, Guarro J. Antifungal susceptibilities of the species of the Pseudallescheria boydii complex. Antimicrob Agents Chemother. 2006;50(12):4211–3.

55. Skiada A, Lanternier F, Groll AH, Pagano L, Zimmerli S, Herbrecht R, et al. Diagnosis and treatment of mucormycosis in patients with hematological malignancies: guidelines from the 3rd European Conference on Infections in Leukemia (ECIL 3). Haematologica. 2013;98(4):492–504.
56. Mantadakis E, Samonis G. Clinical presentation of zygomycosis. Clin Microbiol Infect. 2009;15(Suppl 5):15–20.
57. Downie ML, Alghounaim M, Davidge KM, Yau Y, Walsh TJ, Pope E, et al. Isolated cutaneous mucormycosis in a pediatric renal transplant recipient. Pediatr Transplant. 2018;22(4):e13172.
58. Nayagam LS, Vijayanand B, Balasubramanian S. Isolated renal mucormycosis in an immunocompetent child. Indian J Nephrol. 2014;24(5):321–3.
59. Roden MM, Zaoutis TE, Buchanan WL, Knudsen TA, Sarkisova TA, Schaufele RL, et al. Epidemiology and outcome of zygomycosis: a review of 929 reported cases. Clin Infect Dis. 2005;41(5):634–53.
60. Kontoyiannis DP, Wessel VC, Bodey GP, Rolston KV. Zygomycosis in the 1990s in a tertiary-care cancer center. Clin Infect Dis. 2000;30(6):851–6.
61. Kauffman CA, Malani AN. Zygomycosis: an emerging fungal infection with new options for management. Curr Infect Dis Rep. 2007;9(6):435–40.
62. Trifilio SM, Bennett CL, Yarnold PR, McKoy JM, Parada J, Mehta J, et al. Breakthrough zygomycosis after voriconazole administration among patients with hematologic malignancies who receive hematopoietic stem-cell transplants or intensive chemotherapy. Bone Marrow Transplant. 2007;39(7):425–9.
63. Lanternier F, Dannaoui E, Morizot G, Elie C, Garcia-Hermoso D, Huerre M, et al. A global analysis of mucormycosis in France: the RetroZygo Study (2005-2007). Clin Infect Dis. 2012;54(Suppl 1):S35–43.
64. Harril WC, Stewart MG, Lee AG, Cernoch P. Chronic rhinocerebral mucormycosis. Laryngoscope. 1996;106(10):1292–7.
65. Castrejon-Perez AD, Welsh EC, Miranda I, Ocampo-Candiani J, Welsh O. Cutaneous mucormycosis. An Bras Dermatol. 2017;92(3):304–11.
66. Tissot F, Agrawal S, Pagano L, Petrikkos G, Groll AH, Skiada A, et al. ECIL-6 guidelines for the treatment of invasive candidiasis, aspergillosis and mucormycosis in leukemia and hematopoietic stem cell transplant patients. Haematologica. 2017;102(3):433–44.
67. van Burik JA, Hare RS, Solomon HF, Corrado ML, Kontoyiannis DP. Posaconazole is effective as salvage therapy in zygomycosis: a retrospective summary of 91 cases. Clin Infect Dis. 2006;42(7):e61–5.
68. Marty FM, Ostrosky-Zeichner L, Cornely OA, Mullane KM, Perfect JR, Thompson GR 3rd, et al. Isavuconazole treatment for mucormycosis: a single-arm open-label trial and case-control analysis. Lancet Infect Dis. 2016;16(7):828–37.
69. Abidi MZ, Sohail MR, Cummins N, Wilhelm M, Wengenack N, Brumble L, et al. Stability in the cumulative incidence, severity and mortality of 101 cases of invasive mucormycosis in high-risk patients from 1995 to 2011: a comparison of eras immediately before and after the availability of voriconazole and echinocandin-amphotericin combination therapies. Mycoses. 2014;57(11):687–98.
70. Kyvernitakis A, Torres HA, Jiang Y, Chamilos G, Lewis RE, Kontoyiannis DP. Initial use of combination treatment does not impact survival of 106 patients with haematologic malignancies and mucormycosis: a propensity score analysis. Clin Microbiol Infect: Off Publ Eur Soc Clin Microbiol Infect Dis. 2016;22(9):811.e1–8.
71. Schieffelin JS, Garcia-Diaz JB, Loss GE Jr, Beckman EN, Keller RA, Staffeld-Coit C, et al. Phaeohyphomycosis fungal infections in solid organ transplant recipients: clinical presentation, pathology, and treatment. Transpl Infect Dis: Off J Transplant Soc. 2014;16(2):270–8.
72. McCarty TP, Baddley JW, Walsh TJ, Alexander BD, Kontoyiannis DP, Perl TM, et al. Phaeohyphomycosis in transplant recipients: results from the transplant associated infection surveillance network (TRANSNET). Med Mycol. 2015;53(5):440–6.
73. Revankar SG, Patterson JE, Sutton DA, Pullen R, Rinaldi MG. Disseminated phaeohyphomycosis: review of an emerging mycosis. Clin Infect Dis. 2002;34(4):467–76.

Neutropenic Fever

Aliyah Baluch and Sarah Shewayish

Abstract Neutropenia is defined as an abnormally low absolute neutrophil count (ANC) and can be further delineated as severe or profound (see below). Recipients of chemotherapy will often have a decreased ANC leading to an increased risk of infections specifically from bacterial sources. Neutropenia traditionally is risk stratified based on duration and depth of neutropenia. Recipients of chemotherapy for acute myelogenous leukemia (AML) and stem cell transplants (SCTs) often are deemed as having high risk neutropenia due to significant depth and duration of neutropenia. The mortality associated with febrile neutropenia is up to 11%, and can be as high as 50% in the setting of severe sepsis or septic shock. By risk stratifying neutropenia and the resultant neutropenic fever, the goal is to decrease the resultant morbidity and mortality (Taplitz et al., J Clin Oncol 36:3043–3054).

Keywords Neutrophil count (ANC) · Severe neutropenia · Profound neutropenia · Neutropenic fever · Drug fever · Chemotherapy induced mucositis · Tumor fever · Transfusion related fever · Graft-versus-host disease · Growth factor · Myeloid reconstitution syndrome · Engraftment syndrome

Background Definitions [1]

- Neutropenia is defined as an absolute neutrophil count (ANC) <1000 μL (equivalent to $<1.0 \times 10^{9}$ /L)
- Severe neutropenia is an ANC <500/μL (equivalent to $<0.5 \times 10^{9}$/L)
- Profound neutropenia is an ANC <100/μL (equivalent to $<0.1 \times 10^{9}$/L)
- High risk neutropenia is neutropenia lasting ≥7 days

A. Baluch, MD, MSc (✉)
Moffitt Cancer Center, Tampa, FL, USA
e-mail: aliyah.baluch@moffitt.org

S. Shewayish, MD
University of South Florida, Tampa, FL, USA

A. P. Velez et al. (eds.), *Infections in Neutropenic Cancer Patients*,
https://doi.org/10.1007/978-3-030-21859-1_8

- Fever in neutropenic patients is defined as a single oral temperature of ≥38.3 °C (101 °F) or a temperature of ≥38.0 °C (100.4 °F) sustained over a 1 h period.

Neutropenic Fever (NPF)

Two categories of neutropenic fevers have been described. Microbiologically-based NPF infection is defined when the cultures isolate an organism. On the other hand clinically documented NPF is present when there is a high clinical suspicion for infection based on physical examination findings or radiological testing but there is a negative microbiologic work up. During the work up of NPF, an infectious origin can be identified either microbiologically and/or clinically in only 30–50% of the cases [2]. This is often related to an incomplete medical exam or untimely collection of specimens such as biopsies or aspirations due to concomitant thrombocytopenia. These patients tend to improve after empiric antibiotic therapy which suggests an occult infection. However other non-infectious causes of fever such as chemotherapy induced mucositis, tumor fever, transfusion related fever, drug fever, or graft-versus-host disease should also be considered as potential causes of unexplained fever [3]. Tumor fever is in part thought to be related to cytokine release by the cancer cells, and it is usually a diagnosis of exclusion. Drug fever is not uncommon particularly from certain chemotherapies or growth factors. A thorough detail orientated history, medication reconciliation and physical exam is important in identifying patterns between medications and fever curves. Drug fever should be suspected in the presence of rash, peripheral eosinophilia and increasing transaminases. These associated symptoms are not always present.

Mucositis is a common cause of neutropenic fever. It often develops when there is an ongoing mucosal barrier injury that results from the toxic effects of chemotherapy allowing for either micro- or macro-translocation of bacterial organisms from the GI tract into the systemic system. Micro-translocation leads mainly to an inflammatory syndrome with negative blood cultures but punctuated with NPF whereas macro-translocation presents with positive blood cultures. Chemotherapy induced mucositis and less frequently radiation induced mucositis can involve the entire gastrointestinal tract including the oral cavity. Studies have shown that it may be more important as a cause of infection than neutropenia itself in cancer patients [4].

Other noninfectious causes of fever not to be overlooked include venous thromboembolism, pulmonary emboli, adrenal insufficiency and stroke. Microbiologically documented infections include catheter associated bacteremia, bacterial translocation from the gastrointestinal, genitourinary or respiratory tract, or from skin and soft tissue infections [2].

When evaluating a patient with neutropenic fever, myeloid reconstitution syndrome and engraftment syndrome are two other phenomena that should be taken into consideration. Myeloid reconstitution syndrome is similar to immune reconstitution syndrome seen in HIV patients after initiation of antiretroviral therapy (ART). With the addition of ART, there is a shift from an immunosuppressed state to a pro-inflammatory state. In the setting of hematological malignancies, it occurs within 15 days of neutrophil recovery and manifests as fevers. Superinfection needs to be ruled out in these circumstances prior to considering discontinuing antimicrobials [5]. Engraftment syndrome, more commonly seen in patients undergoing autologous stem cell transplants than SCT, develop fevers, rash and pulmonary infiltrates at the beginning of engraftment; i.e. neutrophil recovery. If the patient has an aggressive and symptomatic engraftment syndrome, steroids can be considered. Patients with breast cancer, previous monotherapy and recent use of G- CSF appear to have higher risk for this syndrome [6].

Microbiology

The causes of bloodstream infection causing neutropenic fever have changed with the use of indwelling catheters and the evolution of chemotherapy modalities. There has been an increased frequency in bacteremias with gram-negative organisms compared to gram positive, with *Enterobacteriaceae* sp. being more predominant, followed by *P. aeruginosa* and other gram negatives. Unfortunately, the use of prophylactic antibiotics has led to an increase in frequency of resistant pathogens such as extended spectrum beta-lactamase (ESBL) producing *Enterobacteriaceae* and carbapenem resistant pathogens. Gram positive bacteria continue to be an important cause of bacteremia. *Staphylococcus aureus* including Methicillin resistant *Staphylococcus aureus* (MRSA), coagulase negative staphylococcus, viridans group streptococcus and *Enterococci*, especially vancomycin resistant *Enterococcus* (VRE) are particularly concerning [2]. Anaerobic bacteria are not as common but have been associated with a polymicrobial bacteremia and in those patients undergoing abdominal surgery. Fungal infections are less common compared to bacterial infections as the cause of fever early in the course of neutropenia. When they are identified, *Aspergillus* sp. and *Candida* sp. are the most common. Non *C. albicans* strains are increasing in frequency due to selective pressure from the ongoing use of prophylactic fluconazole [2]. The greatest risk factor for mold infection is profound and prolonged neutropenia (i.e. 14 days or more with ANC < 100).

Management

Management for neutropenic fever first starts with a discussion of appropriate prophylaxis which has been risk stratified on the basis of the anticipated duration of neutropenia [1]. The optimal time to choose a patient's regimen for a future neutropenic fever is during the initial consult by an infectious diseases consultant after discussing all of the risk stratifying past medical issues for a particular patient including but not limited to previous infections especially while neutropenic. In addition, prophylaxis against *Pseudomonas* and other Enterobacteriaceae are of outmost importance in this population. Unfortunately, *Pseudomonas* continues to be a significant cause for neutropenic fever. Other enteric gram-negative rods (GNRs) are important sources of bacteremia after chemotherapy induced mucosal damage resulting in mucositis/enteritis and bacterial translocation [2].

Risk Factors for Febrile Neutropenia

The risk of febrile neutropenia not only depends on the duration and degree of neutropenia but also on other factors related to the demographics of the patient, for example the malignancy in question or the treatment regimen being delievered [1]. The highest risk for NPF is in in patients with profound and protracted neutropenia after induction chemotherapy for acute leukemia and in the pre-engraftment stage following SCT infusion Table 1. Summarizes key risk factors.

Primary Prophylaxis

In terms of antimicrobial prophylaxis there is a three-pronged approach. The first prong is antibacterial. The second is antifungal and the third is antiviral [1]. Traditionally antibacterial prophylaxis is utilized to prevent first and foremost an invasive *Pseudomonas* (PSA) infection, thus the use of ciprofloxacin or levofloxacin.

Table 1 Common Risk Factors for Neutropenic Fever

Factors related to	Higher risk
Patient factors/ characteristics	Advanced age
	Low performance status
	Low albumin
	Prior episode of neutropenia
	Presence of comorbidities
Malignancy	Acute leukemia
	Myelodysplastic syndrome (MDS)
	High grade lymphoma
	Soft tissue sarcoma
	Non Hodgkin Lymphoma (NHL)/myeloma
	Increased risk if advanced stage or not in remission or if in relapse
Treatment regimen	High doses of anthracyclines, cisplatin, ifosfamide, cyclophosphamide, etoposide or cytarabine
	Remission-induction and rescue chemotherapy
	Duration and degree of GI/oral mucositis

Levofloxacin is the best choice if there is a concomitant need for viridans group streptococcus (VGS) due to dental or gingival issues. If a patient has prolonged QT corrected or is intolerant of a fluoroquinolone, the alternative option for antibacterial prophylaxis is cefdinir or cefpodoxime [1]. Unfortunately, with this approach, there is an increased risk for pseudomonas bacteremia due to the lack of coverage with oral cephalosporins. Primary prophylaxis is recommended for patients who are at high risk for febrile neutropenia or with profound and protracted neutropenia (ANC ≤100 for >7 days), such as patients with AML/MDS or SCT treated with myeloablative conditioning regimens. Current guidelines do not recommend routine prophylaxis in patients with low risk neutropenia such as those with solid tumors [1, 7]. Due to the increase of multidrug resistant organisms (MDROs) there are regions of the world including the northeast of the US where the rates are higher for drug resistance for PSA as well as other gram-negative rods (GNRs) making the use of antibacterial prophylaxis useless and only increases the risk of *Clostridium difficile* infection (CDI) (Tables 2 and 3).

For primary antifungal prophylaxis, the drug of choice depends on the total assessment of the patient's current situation (disease status, chemotherapy present and past, if there is a history of fungal infections, and potential lifetime exposures). It is important to risk stratify to adequately estimate the pre-test probability of invasive yeast infection versus mold infection in neutropenic patients. For example, an acute myelogenous leukemia (AML) undergoing induction chemotherapy would be a candidate for voriconazole primary prophylaxis due to the risk of neutropenia in a patient expecting neutropenic longer than 14 days (a known risk factor for invasive mold infection). Prophylaxis against invasive *Aspergillus* sp. infections with posaconazole is considered for patients ≥13 years of age, and undergoing intense chemotherapy for AML or MDS [1]. On the other hand, an impending neutropenic patient for SCT may have duration of neutropenia less than 14 days thus fluconazole or an echinocandin would be sufficient for prophylaxis against *Candida* sp. Antifungal prophylaxis is recommended for patients expected to have profound, protracted neutropenia such as patients with AML/MDS or SCT patients [1]. Similar

Table 2 Non-infectious causes of fever in cancer patients

Mucositis
Graft versus host disease (GVHD)
Myeloid reconstitution syndrome
Pre-engraftment syndrome
Drug fever
Tumor fever
Deep venous thrombosis (DVTs), thromboembolism
Stroke
Transfusion-related fevers
Fever secondary to G-CSF/ GM-CSF
Radiation-related fevers

Table 3 Microbiology of infections in febrile neutropenia

Bacterial	Gram negative pathogens (blood stream infections)
	Enterobacteriaceae, 24%
	P. aeruginosa, 10%
	Acinetobacter, 2%
	Other gram negatives, 3%
	Gram positive pathogens (blood stream infections)
	S. aureus, 6%
	Coagulase-negative staphylococci, 25%
	Viridans group streptococci, 5%
	Enterococci, 5%
	Other gram positives, 6%
	Clostridium difficile (GI infections)
	Helicobacter pylori (GI infections)
	Salmonella and *Shigella* (rare)
	Mycoplasma pneumoniae (pulmonary infections)
	Chlamydia pneumoniae (pulmonary infections)
	Tuberculosis
Fungal	Candida spp.
	P. *jirovecii*
	Cryptococci
	Aspergillus spp.
	Mucorales
	Fusarium
	Scedosporium
Viral	Herpes simplex virus (reactivation in 60% HSV sero-positive)
	Hepatitis B virus and hepatitis C virus reactivation)
	Cytomegalovirus (CMV)
	Respiratory syncytial virus (RSV)
	Influenza A or B
	Parainfluenza 1–4
	Metapneumovirus
	Adenoviruses
	Coronaviruses
	Rhinoviruses/Enterovirus
	Norovirus
Other Pathogens	Strongyloidiasis
	Leishmaniasis, trypanosomiasis, malaria

to antibacterial prophylaxis, anti-mold prophylaxis is not recommended for solid tumors. Regimens associated with an increased risk of infection by *Pneumocystis jirovecii* such as those patients on purine analogues or those on ≥20 mg of prednisone for more than 1 month should receive trimethoprim-sulfamethoxazole ideally in daily dosing to increase compliance. If intolerant or allergic to trimethoprim-

Table 4 MASCC scoring system to identify patients with cancer and FN at low risk of medical complications

Burden of FN with no or mild symptoms	5
No hypotension	5
No COPD	4
Solid tumor or hematological malignancy with no previous fungal infection	4
No dehydration requiring IV fluids	3
Burden of FN with moderate symptoms	3
Outpatient status	3
Age < 60	2
Maximum score is 26, ≥ 21 low risk	

Table 5 The clinical index of stable febrile neutropenia (CISNE)

Explanatory Variable	
Eastern Cooperative Oncology Group performance status ≥ 2	2
COPD	1
Chronic cardiovascular disease	1
National Cancer Institute common toxicity criteria mucositis of grade ≥ 2	1
Monocytes <200 μL	1
Stress-induced hyperglycemia	2

0–8 score. Low risk (zero points), intermediate risk (1–2 points), high risk (≥3 points)

sulfamethoxazole then alternatives such as dapsone, atovaquone or aerosolized pentamidine can be considered [1]. Prior to utilizing dapsone, ensuring the patient has a sufficient level of G6PD is recommended.

As far as antiviral prophylaxis, HSV seropositive patients undergoing leukemia induction therapy or SCT should receive prophylaxis. In terms of primary herpes simplex or varicella prophylaxis, traditionally acyclovir at either 400 mg BID by mouth or 800 mg BID by mouth is utilized. Per specific indications like previous breakthrough infections while on acyclovir, a patient may be considered a candidate for a pro-drug such as famciclovir or valacyclovir for prophylaxis while neutropenic. Tenofovir or entecavir is recommended for patients whom are at risk of hepatitis B reactivation while on chemotherapy or immunotherapy that is B-cell depleting [1, 2] (Tables 4 and 5).

Secondary Prophylaxis

When evaluating the patient for impending neutropenia, the infectious diseases (ID) team needs to review the patient's medical history. In general if a particular infection develops while neutropenic, there is a concern that the patient will be at risk for reactivation/recurrence of the same infection when creating the same situation again i.e. a new episode of neutropenia. The drug(s) that was (were) used to treat the original infection should be re-considered as the ideal drug to resume when the patient becomes neutropenic during subsequent episodes. By creating the same milieu that lead to the infection in the first place, the patient is now at risk for that infection to recur. For example, if voriconazole was used to treat a fungal pneumonia during induction chemotherapy, one should consider restarting voriconazole for secondary prophylaxis for the impending neutropenia expected during SCT [1, 8].

Other Considerations

The role of granulocyte colony stimulating factor (G-CSF) in prophylaxis is at times controversial. G-CSF has shown to decrease length and degree of neutropenia and reduce the risk of febrile neutropenia in solid tumors however it has not shown to decrease the risk of febrile neutropenia or reduce mortality in hematological malignancies. The recommendation overall is to give G-CSF in patients who are on chemotherapy regimens known to have a 20% increase risk of febrile neutropenia or in presence of comorbidities but lower risk [7].

Hand hygiene, diet and other environmental factors are also to be considered. It is recommended to avoid undercooked meats, unpasteurized milk, unpasteurized cheese or unpeeled fruits and vegetables unless washed properly at home [1, 2]. Also, neutropenic patients in an outpatient setting should avoid contact with environments that have high concentrations of airborne fungal spores such as construction/renovation sites, intense gardening and digging [1, 2]. In the same line of thinking of minimizing exposure to plant matter, it is not recommended for neutropenic or impending neutropenic patients to utilize tobacco products or marijuana products due to the theoretical risk of fungal pneumonia.

Outpatient Versus Inpatient Therapy

The management of neutropenic patients who present with fever can be divided into inpatient versus outpatient management. It is also important to identify patients presenting to the outpatient setting who will require inpatient referral [1] (Tables 6 and 7).

When a cancer patient with fever and neutropenia comes to an emergency room for evaluation, it should be assumed that there is an infectious cause until proven otherwise. Per the 2010 IDSA clinical guidelines, an assessment should be done within 15 min of being seen in triage. A complete history and physical as well as appropriate lab work including a complete blood count (CBC), renal function test, lactic acid level, and liver function test should be performed. Blood cultures should

Table 6 Talcott's rules

Group	Characteristic
I	Inpatients (at time of fever onset)
II	Outpatients with acute comorbidity requiring hospitalization
III	Outpatients without comorbidity but with no uncontrolled cancer
IV	Outpatients with controlled cancer and without comorbidity

Group IV is low risk

Table 7 Spectrum of antimicrobial activity in neutropenic fever

	Pseudomonas coverage	Anaerobic coverage	Enterococcal coverage	ESBL coverage
Anti-Pseudomonal cephalosporin (i.e. cefepime)	+	–	–	–
Pip-tazo	+	+	++	±
Anti-Pseudomonal carbapenem (i.e. meropenem)	+	+	+	+

be collected from different sites including a peripheral stick as well as a culture from each of the lumens of a patient's central catheter if present. Other cultures such as urine, CSF and imaging such as a chest x-ray are obtained as clinically indicated. Patents with influenza-like symptoms should be tested for influenza ideally via polymerase chain reactions (PCR). Empiric antimicrobial therapy should be administered within 1 h from presentation to the ER [1]. Either an antipseudomonal B-lactam or a carbapenem should be given empirically for NPF. Additional gram-positive coverage is recommended only when there is suspicion of a gram-positive producing infection such as line infection or soft tissue infection where the addition of IV vancomycin is indicated [1]. Empiric NPF regimens are designed to be adjusted based on patient risk factors i.e. known ESBL colonization and the need for empiric meropenem. Traditionally if the patient is colonized with MRSA, there is the consideration of empiric 48 h use of IV vancomycin, linezolid or daptomycin. If the patient is colonized with vancomycin resistant enterococcus (VRE) then there is a consideration of 48 h of empiric daptomycin or linezolid use for NPF. Carbapenamase producing organisms in a patient's history would lead the ID team to consider the early use of prolonged infusion meropenem and polymyxin-colistin or ceftazidime avibactam if sensitive in the past. Anaerobic coverage is added as clinically indicated [10].

If a NPF develops on the outpatient service, the decision algorithm has to assess the need for inpatient versus outpatient care. Febrile neutropenia in patients who are expected to be neutropenic for more than 7 days and have profound neutropenia and/or have significant comorbidities is deemed high risk. These patients are then candidates for inpatient therapy [1]. On the other hand, patients with febrile neutropenia who are expected to have a short duration of neutropenia and none/few comorbidities would therefore be considered low risk. Low risk patients are then considered candidates for outpatient therapy. There are several tools that have been validated to supplement clinical decision making: MASCC index, Talcott's rules or CISNE (specifically for solid tumors presenting with NPF). These tools are designed to augment clinical decision making but if the patient is deemed unstable for discharge by a treating physician from an emergency room then regardless of the score, the patient would need admission to the hospital [8]. Also those patients infected with a resistant pathogen will have a higher pretest probability of admission due to the difficulty in organizing intravenous antimicrobials from an emergency room setting. Afebrile patients who have new signs or symptoms suggestive of an infection that are considered high-risk would automatically be candidates for inpatient therapy [2, 7].

If the patient is determined to be stable for outpatient management, after also taking into consideration logistic factors such as ease of follow up visits, and transportation, among others then they can be discharged after 4 h of the initial hospital, ER or clinic assessment. Empiric therapy for NPF on the outpatient service would be an oral fluoroquinolone plus amoxicillin-clavulanate acid or clindamycin (if the patient was penicillin allergic) [1]. If these patients were previously on an oral fluoroquinolone for prophylaxis then they should not be given empiric therapy with a fluoroquinolone. Prior prophylaxis with a fluoroquinolone followed by NPF is an indication to be admitted to an inpatient unit until a resistant bacterial infection is rule out. If a patient fails to defervesce after 2–3 days or he/she develops a new NPF, new infection or if initial blood cultures become positive or intolerance to oral therapy develops, then reevaluation and hospital admission is indicated [1, 7].

Tailoring therapy depends on the individual's clinical course. Patients with unexplained fevers but who are stable would be continued on the initial therapy for up to 5 days prior to consideration for either a lateral change (possible drug fever) versus escalation (concern for inadequate coverage) ± CT chest without contrast to rule out an occult mold infection. If the patient has a documented infection then the antimicrobial regimen should be adjusted to reflect the positive cultures. Those patients who are on IV therapy can also be switched at that point to oral therapy if GI absorption is deemed adequate and they are clinically stable. Those patients who become unstable or hypotensive, should have their regimen broadened to cover for resistant pathogens [1, 7]. With persistent NPF beyond 5 days, the consideration needs to be made for empirically adjusting antifungal coverage to include anti-mold therapy. Antiviral therapy is indicated in febrile neutropenia only if there is strong clinical or laboratory evidence of a viral infection. If there is an ongoing community-based outbreak of influenza A or B, then a febrile neutropenic patient presenting with influenza-like symptoms should be treated empirically with neuraminidase inhibitors [1, 7].

When to De-escelate Therapy?

This topic used to be controversial when it comes to NPF but there is an increasing breadth of knowledge and guidelines to support de-escalation under the auspices of antimicrobial stewardship. Per 2010 IDSA clinical guidelines, it depends on the duration of neutropenia as well as having a clinically or microbiologically documented infection [1]. In the setting of an unexplained fever, the initial therapy should be continued until there is marrow recovery i.e. ANC >500. In the case of a documented infection, therapy depends on the site of infection and or organism isolated. Antibiotics (whether prophylaxis or treatment) are continued until the ANC > 500 or if they received an appropriate duration of therapy for that particular infection, then they can be switched to prophylactic antibiotics for the remaining duration of neutropenia [1]. However there have been an increasing collection of studies and the European Guidelines that recommend early de-escalation of antibiotics back to prophylaxis in cases of resolved unexplained fever. When considering this option, patients should be afebrile at least for >48 h, clinically stable, and without signs or symptoms of new infection [9].

Pathogen Based Treatment Algorithms

With the advent of multiplex polymerase chain reactions (PCRs), the paradigm of treating neutropenic fever is slowly but steadily changing. Multiple microbiology labs have invested into an array of platforms that help facilitate the rapid diagnosis of bacteremias. The previous paradigm was monitoring blood cultures continuously for up to 5 days or at least until they turned positive. Once the blood culture turned positive, an initial sample was assessed via a gram stain. Simultaneously the sample is plated with the goal of growing a pure colony to run through a VITEK II allowing for the assessment of antimicrobial sensitivities as well as placing a sample in one of many types of PCR platforms. Based on the example of the BioFire©, the turnaround time for the blood culture identification (BCID) panel is approximately 1 h. after only 5 min of hands on time. This allows for the identification of the organism but unfortunately for sensitivities, one still has to wait for the pure culture to be selected out and run through the VITEK II [11]. The integration of matrix-assisted laser desorption/ionization time-of-flight mass spectrometry (MALDI-TOF MS) has further changed the face of microbiology by utilizing protein fingerprinting to diagnose organisms by use of referencing them against a database and various algorithms [12].

Key Points

- Neutropenic fever among cancer patients may be associated with significant morbidity and mortality.
- Prophylaxis is indicated for patients with profound, protracted neutropenia to reduce the risk of febrile episodes related to infection.
- All cancer patients who are neutropenic, presenting with fever should be evaluated for infection while also ruling out other non-infectious causes of fever.
- Thorough evaluation augmented by clinical judgment and if needed specific scoring tools should be implemented to identify those patients with febrile neutropenia who require inpatient management.
- Empiric antimicrobial therapy involves the use of antibiotics with anti-pseudomonal coverage, with the addition of gram-positive coverage depending on the clinical scenario.
- Antifungal coverage and the evaluation of fungal infections in high risk patients should be considered with profound neutropenia with persistent fevers.
- Timing of de-escalation of therapy is still debatable however for stable patients with resolved, unexplained fevers after 48 h of therapy can be de-escalated back to prophylaxis and followed closely if clinically stable.

References

1. Taplitz R, A, Kennedy EB, Bow EJ, Crews J, Gleason C, Hawley DK, Langston AA, Nastoupil LJ, Rajotte M, Rolston KV, Strasfeld L, Flowers CR. Antimicrobial prophylaxis for adult patients with cancer- related immunosuppression: ASCO and IDSA clinical practice guideline update. J Clin Oncol. 36:3043–54. © 2018 by American Society of Clinical Oncology
2. Bennett, JE. Mandell, Douglas, and Bennett's principles and practice of infectious diseases. 8th ed: Elsevier, Philadelphia, US
3. Pasikhova Y, Ludlow S, Baluch A. Fever in patients with cancer. Cancer Cont J Moffit Cancer Center. 2017;24(2)
4. van der Velden WJFM, Herbers AHE, Netea MG, Blijlevens NMA. Mucosal barrier injury, fever and infection in neutropenic patients with cancer: introducing the paradigm febrile mucositis. John Wiley & Sons Ltd Br J Haematol. 2014;167:441–52.
5. Bhagavath A, Geyer A. Memorial sloan kettering. New York. CHEST Annual Meeting 2016 Los Angeles October 22–26
6. Akasheh M, Eastwood D, Vesole DH. Engraftment syndrome after autologous hematopoietic stem cell transplant supported by granulocyte-colony-stimulating factor (G-CSF) versus granulocyte-macrophage colony-stimulating factor (GM-CSF). Bone Marrow Transplant. 2003;31:113–6.
7. Freifeld AG, Bow EJ, Sepkowitz KA, Boeckh MJ, Ito JI, Mullen CA, et al. Clinical practice guideline for the use of antimicrobial agents in neutropenic patients with cancer: 2010 update by the infectious diseases society of america. Clin Infect Dis. 2011;52(4):e56–93.
8. Taplitz RA, Kennedy EB, Bow EJ, Crews J, Gleason C, Hawley DK, Langston AA, Nastoupil LJ, Rajotte M, Rolston K, Strasfeld L, Flowers CR. Outpatient management of fever and neutropenia in adults treated for malignancy: American Society of Clinical Oncology and

Infectious Diseases Society of America clinical practice guideline update. J Clin Oncol. 2018 May 10;36(14):1443–53. https://doi.org/10.1200/JCO.2017.6211.
9. Le Clech L, Talarmin J-P, Couturier M-A, Ianotto J-C, Nicol C, Le Calloch R, Santos SD, Hutin P, DidierTandé VC, Berthou C, Guillerm G. Early discontinuation of empirical antibacterial therapy in febrile neutropenia: the ANTIBIOSTOP study. Infect Dis. 2018;50(7):539–49. https://doi.org/10.1080/23744235.2018.1438649.
10. Rosa RG, dos Santos RP, Goldani LZ. Comparison of anti-anaerobic antimicrobial strategies in cancer patients with febrile neutropenia and gastrointestinal symptoms. BMC Res Notes. 2014;7:614.
11. Altun O, Almuhayawi M, Ullberg M, Ozenci V. Clinical evaluation of the FilmArray blood culture identification panel in identification of bacteria and yeasts from positive blood culture bottles. J Clin Microbiol. 2013;51(12):4130–6.
12. Lee AWT, Lam JKS, Lam RKW, Ng WH, Lee ENL, Lee VTY, et al. Comprehensive evaluation of the MBT STAR-BL module for simultaneous bacterial identification and beta-lactamase-mediated resistance detection in gram-negative rods from cultured isolates and positive blood cultures. Front Microbiol. 2018;9:334.

Antifungal Medications in Neutropenia

Rod Quilitz

Abstract Over the last two decades, clinicians managing invasive fungal infections in neutropenic cancer patients have encountered many challenges – please see chapter on "Fungal Infections". Fortunately we have also seen an expansion in our antifungal armamentarium during this time frame as well. This chapter will focus on the antifungal agents which are utilized for the prevention and treatment of invasive fungal infections in the neutropenic cancer patient. Specifically, we will discuss the polyene antifungal amphotericin B, the anti-metabolite flucytosine, select azole antifungals (fluconazole, voriconazole, posaconazole, isavuconazonium sulfate), and the echinocandins (caspofungin, micafungin, anidulafungin).

Keywords Polyene Antifungals · Amphotericin B deoxycholate · Nystatin · Flucytosine · Azole antifungal · Fluconazole · Voriconazole · Posaconazole · Isavuconazonium sulfate · Echinocandin Antifungals · Caspofungin · Micafungin

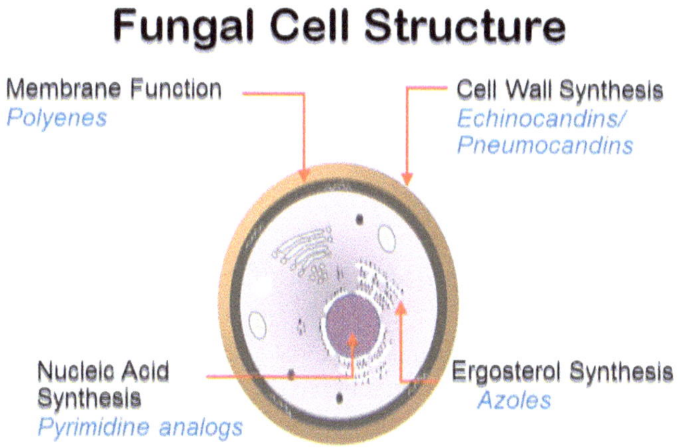

R. Quilitz, PharmD, BCOP (✉)
Infectious Diseases and Antimicrobial Stewardship, Moffitt Cancer Center, Tampa, FL, USA
e-mail: Rod.Quilitz@moffitt.org

A. P. Velez et al. (eds.), *Infections in Neutropenic Cancer Patients*,
https://doi.org/10.1007/978-3-030-21859-1_9

Polyene Antifungals

Amphotericin B

Stucture of Amphotericin B [1]

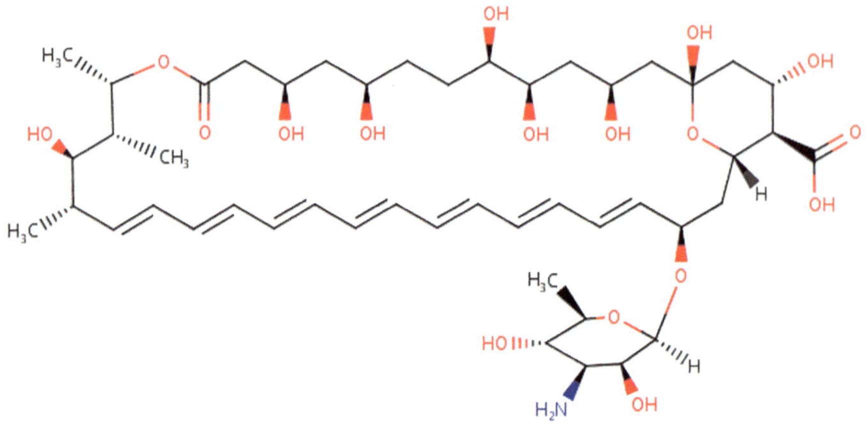

Amphotericin B deoxycholate (Fungizone, AmBD), also known as "conventional" amphotericin B, is a broad-spectrum, fungicidal polyene antifungal agent which was a life-saving innovative agent when it was FDA approved in 1959 [2]. Amphoterin B binds to ergosterol on the fungal cell membrane then merges into the fungal cell membrane causing a pore which allows for increased passage of fluids into the fungal cell and cell rupture [1–3]. Amphotericin B deoxycholate was the primary agent for the treatment of invasive fungal infections for decades but its use was limited by its toxicity which lead to the development of lipid formulations of amphotericin B which have largely replaced the use of AmBD in the neutropenic cancer patient population [2].

Amphotericin B Antifungal Spectrum of Activity

Amphotericin B has broad-spectrum fungicidal activity for a wide variety of invasive fungal infections including but not limited to aspergillosis, candidiasis, fusariosis, mucormycosis, and the endemic mycosis such as blastomycosis, histoplasmosis, coccidiomycosis, paracoccidioidomycois, and sporotrichosis [3, 4]. Amphotericin B resistance is typically associated with a MIC >2 mg/L [4] and has been most commonly reported in *Candida lusitanie* [4], *Aspergillus terreus* [5], *Scedosporium* species [4], and *Trichosporin beigelii* [6]. More recently, there are increasing reports of amphotericin B resistance among some isolates of *Candida auris* [7] and *Fusarium* [8].

Amphotericin B Adverse Reactions

Conventional amphotericin B has been referred to by clinicians and sometimes patients as "Ampho-terrible" due to the frequency of infusion reactions and nephrotoxicity [2].

Amphotericin B associated infusion reactions, sometimes known unofficially as the "Shake and Bake Syndrome," can cause fevers, chills, and rigors but also nausea and vomiting, headache, arthralgias, myalgias, and ever anaphylactoid reactions resulting in acute dyspnea [2, 3, 9]. Pre-medications such as hydrocortisone (50 mg PO/IV), acetaminophen (650 mg PO), and diphenhydramine (25–50 mg PO/IV) may reduce the incidence and severity of these reactions although quality clinical trial data is lacking [9]. Amphotericin B induced rigors have been treated with opioids such as hydromorphone (0.5 mg IV) or meperidine (25 mg IV), typically allowing for completion of the amphotericin B infusion [2, 9]. One study which randomized patients to receive AmBD over 4 versus 24 h per day demonstrated a more than 50% reduction in the incidence of fever, chills, and rigors with the extended infusion [10].

Amphotericin B induced nephrotoxicity risk increases with cumulative dose and can result in an acute decline in glomerular filtration rate with associated rise in serum creatinine as well as urinary wasting of potassium and magnesium [2, 9]. Saline loading (NS 500 mL IV before and after each dose) may reduce or delay AmBD nephrotoxicity but does not affect electrolyte wasting [9, 11]. Continuous infusion AmBD has also recently been demonstrated to be less nephrotoxic compared to a 4 h daily IV infusion [10].

Amphotericin B induced hypokalemia and hypomagnesemia can be severe and require close laboratory monitoring throughout therapy – in addition to acute replacement with intravenous and/or oral electrolytes, scheduled oral potassium chloride and/or magnesium oxide supplementation is often required [9]. Amiloride 5–10 mg PO BID can also be utilized to reduce AmBD induced potassium wasting but it should be discontinued with or shortly after the completion of amphotericin B therapy to avoid hyperkalemia as the renal tubules recover [12].

Lipid Formulations of Amphotericin B

Three lipid formulations of amphotericin B were developed to reduce toxicity of this agent while preserving its efficacy: Amphotericin B Lipid Complex (Abelcet, ABLC) FDA approved in 1995, Amphotericin B Cholesterol Sulfate or AmB Colloidal Dispersion (Amphotec, ABCD) FDA approved in 1996, and Liposomal Amphotericin B (Ambisome, L-AmB) FDA approved in 1997 [2].

The lipid formulations were primarily designed to reduce nephrotoxicity and, as expected, all 3 agents have been demonstrated to be less nephrotoxic than AmBD [2, 13]. A randomized, double-blind comparative trial in patients with persistent neutropenic fever by Wingard and colleagues compared ABLC to two doses of L-AmB and demonstrated reduced risk for nephrotoxicity in the L-Amb group (14.1% and 14.8% vs. 42.3%, $P < 0.01$) [14].

Adverse infusion reactions vary by amphotericin B formulation [13]. ABCD has a higher incidence of rate of infusion reactions than AmBD: including chills (53% vs 30%) and fever (27% vs 16%) [15]. Wingard and colleagues demonstrated that L-Amb exhibited a lower rate of chills and rigors than ABLC (18.8% and 23.5% vs 79.5%) on day 1 [14]. While L-Amb appears to have the lowest incidence of infusion-related reactions among the amphotericin B formulations, a minority of patients may experience an atypical hyper-acute and often very dramatic infusion reaction to L-Amb involving one or more of the following adverse effects: " [1] chest pain, dyspnea, and hypoxia [2]; severe abdomen, flank, or leg pain; and/or [3] flushing and urticaria" [16]. In these rare cases of atypical L-Amb infusion reactions, stop the infusion immediately and consider intravenous diphenhydramine. For future doses, high dose intravenous diphenhydramine (up to 1 mg/kg) has been added to pre-medications prior to subsequent doses [16] or, in our experience, many of these patients can tolerate ABLC with aggressive pre-medication and initially reduced rate of infusion.

Due to their superior safety profile and equivalent efficacy, lipid formulations of amphotericin B are preferred over AmBD [2, 13] in the treatment of invasive fungal infections in neutropenic cancer patients. A direct comparison of continuous infusion AmBD to a lipid formulation could be of value.

Amphotericin B Dosing Recommendations

Amphotericin B Deoxycholate (Fungizone) – use actual body weight for dosing in obese patients [17]

Aspergillosis	1–1.5 mg/kg IV Q24H
Blastomycosis	0.7–1 mg/kg IV Q24H, total dose of 2–2.5 g
Candida esophagitis	0.3–0.7 mg/kg IV Q24H
Candidemia or Disseminated Candidasis	0.7–1 mg/kg IV Q24H
Coccidioidomycosis	0.5–0.7 mg/kg IVQ24H, total dose 7–20 mg/kg
Cryptococcal meningitis	0.7 mg/kg IV Q24H in combination with flucytosine for a minimum of 2 weeks and CSF is sterile, then fluconazole
Histoplamsosis	0.7–1 mg/kg IV Q24H
Mucormycosis	1–1.5 mg/kg IV Q24H, total dose of 30–40 mg/kg

Amphotericin B Lipid Complex (Abelcet) – consider ideal body weight for dosing in obese patients [16]	
Invasive Fungal Infections	5 mg/kg IV Q24H
Liposomal Amphotericin B (Ambisome) – consider ideal body weight for dosing in obese patients [16]	
Aspergillosis	3 mg/kg IV Q24H [18] (3 mg/kd/day with same efficacy, less toxicity than 10 mg/kg/day for first 2 weeks of therapy) [18]
Candidemia	3–5 mg/kg IV Q24H
Fusariosis/Mucormycosis	5 mg/kg IV Q24H, higher doses of 10–15 mg/kg/day have been used in refractory infections
Persistent neutropenic fever	3 mg/kg IV Q24H, up to 5 mg/kg IV Q24H
Antifungal prophylaxis in high risk	1 mg/kg IV Q24H [19] or 10 mg/kg IV (over 2 h) weekly [20] or
Neutropenics intolerant to other options	15 mg/kg IV (over 6 h) every other week [21]
Antifungal prophylaxis to reduce the risk Of Invasive Pulmonary Aspergillosis	12.5 mg over 30 min via nebulizer On 2 consecutive days per week [22]

Nystatin

Structure of nystatin [23]

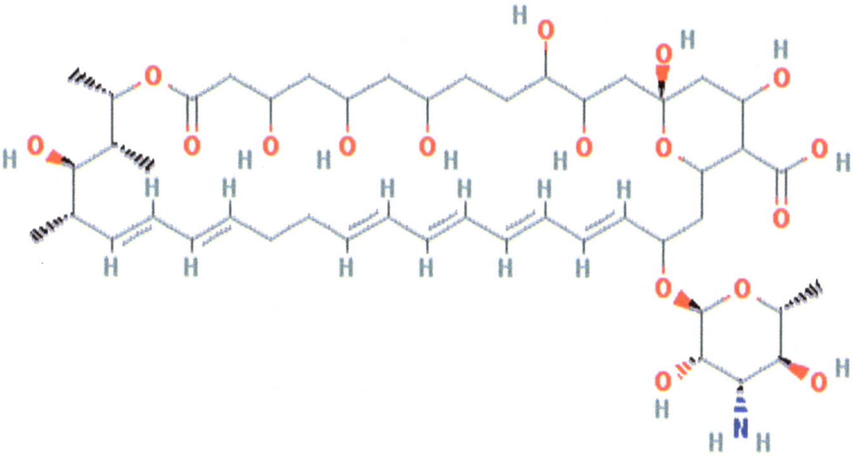

Nystatin (Mycostatin), like amphotericin B, is a polyene antifungal agent which was discovered in 1950 [24]. The antifungal spectrum of nystatin is comparable, but not identical, to that of amphotericin B [24]. Strains of *Candida albicans* have been identified that are much more susceptible to nystatin than amphotericin B [24]. Nystatin may also exhibit activity against *Candida glabrata, Candida krusei, Geotrichum*, and *Beauvaria* which are amphotericin B resistant [24].

Intravenous nystatin was initially investigated for the treatment of invasive fungal infections but it was never FDA approved due to excessive toxicities including venous sclerosis as well as intolerable infusion related infusions such as severe fever, rigors, and malaise [24]. A liposomal formulation of nystatin, with the goal of reducing toxicity, has been studied in phase 1 and 2 studies primarily [24]. Offner and colleagues studied the use of liposomal nystatin in 26 patients with invasive aspergillosis who either could not tolerate amphotericin B or whose infection was refractory to amphotericin B [25]. In this trial of high risk patients, the overall response rate was 28% with 68% overall mortality and a high incidence (67%) of infusion related reactions which lead to discontinuation in 2 patients [25]. Nephrotoxicity and hypokalemia were manageable in this study [25]. Liposomal nystatin has to date not been submitted to the FDA for review and remains unavailable outside of clinical trials.

Due to lack of significant bioavailability, nystatin can be safely administered swish-and-swallow for the treatment of oral candidiasis or topically for the management of cutaneous and vaginal fungal infections, predominantly for candidiasis [24].

Nystatin dosing [26]	
Thrush	500,000–1,000,000 units (5–10 mL) in mouth 35× per day Half of suspension in left side of mouth, swish as long as possible before swallowing, then repeat in right side of mouth.
Cutaneous candidiasis	Apply cream, ointment, or powder to affected areas BID
Vaginal candidiasis	1 vaginal tablet (100,000 units) daily for 2 weeks

Flucytosine

Structure of flucytosine [27]

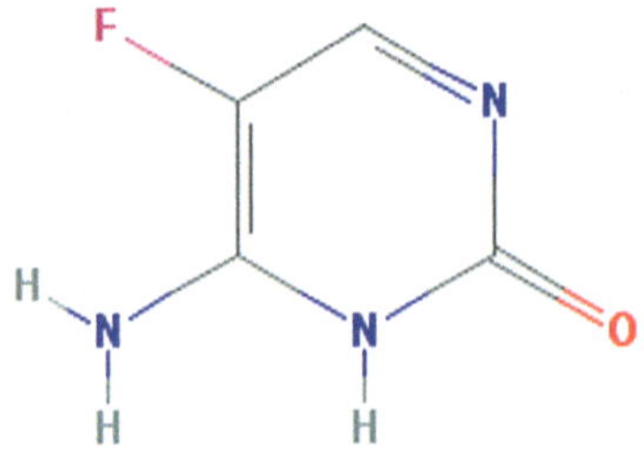

Flucytosine (Ancobon, FC) has been available as 250 mg and 500 mg capsules for oral administration since 1968 [28, 29]. Currently FC is the only antimetabolite agent with antifungal activity. Flucytosine inhibits fungal protein synthesis by replacing uracil with 5-flourouracil (5-FU) in fungal RNA as well as inhibiting thymidylate synthetase via 5- fluorodeoxy-uridine monophosphatase which interferes with fungal DNA synthesis [28, 29].

Flucytosine Antifungal Spectrum of Activity

Flucytosine's activity against yeasts include *Candida* (except for *Candida krusei) and Cryptococcus* [29]. Flucytosine is recommended to be used in combination with amphotericin B (either conventional or lipid formulations) for the treatment of Cryptococcal meningitis due to the enhanced rate of CSF clearance as well as improved survival compared to amphotericin B plus fluconazole 800 mg/day [30]. Flucytosine has been used in combination with amphotericin B or fluconazole in patients with refractory invasive *Candida* infections despite lack of randomized clinical trial data to support this indication [29]. The 2016 Infectious Disease Society of America (IDSA) Candidiasis guidelines note that flucytosine in combination with amphotericin B may be considered for CNS infections, endocarditis, and endopthalmitis [31]. Flucytosine is typically not recommended as monotherapy for invasive yeast infections due to baseline resistance in 7–8% of *Candida* species and rapid induction of resistance [29]. Flucytosine monotherapy may be considered as an option for the treatment of fluconazole-resistant *Candida glabrata* urinary tract infections given the high concentrations achieved in the urinary tract with this renally cleared antifungal agent [29, 31].

Flucytosine has *in vitro* activity against *Aspergillus* species and had been utilized in the pre-echinocandin era as part of combination therapy for refractory cases of aspergillosis despite lack of data to support this practice [29]. Flucytosine is not, however, mentioned in the 2016 IDSA Aspergillosis guidelines [32].

Flucytosine Adverse Reactions and Financial Toxicity

As may be expected for a pro-drug of the cytotoxic cancer agent 5-fluorouracil, flucytosine's most clinically significant adverse effect is myelosuppression [29]. Flucytosine drug induced neutropenia and thrombocytopenia more so than anemia is typically observed within the first 2 weeks of therapy in 27% of patients and is usually associated with FC serum concentrations >100 mg/L [29].

Hepatotoxicity may be a significant complication of FC therapy and has been reported to occur in up to 41% of patients [29]. Most commonly this consists of reversible elevated transaminases and alkaline phosphatase [29]. Hyperbilirubinemia is less common than transaminitis and there have been 2 cases of life-threatening liver necrosis attributed to FC [29]. It may be possible to reduce the incidence of FC induced hepatotoxicity by avoiding peak FC concentrations above 100 mg/L [29].

Gastrointestinal side effects such as nausea and diarrhea more so than vomiting and abdominal pain can occur in approximately 6% of patients receiving FC [29].

Unfortunately, the exorbitant cost of flucytosine in the United States is worthy of mention. In 2009, Valeant Pharmaceuticals acutely increased the price of flucytosine to the extent that a 2 week course of FC costs approximately $28,000 for FC alone whereas the cost in the United Kingdom is one-tenth of this price [33]. While this has resulted in enhanced scrutiny of FC utilization in the United States, even at this inflated price the combination of amphotericin B plus flucytosine may be cost-effective for the treatment of Cryptococcal meningitis given superior efficacy compared to amphotericin B plus high dose fluconazole [33].

Flucytosine Dosing [28, 34] & Therapeutic Drug Monitoring [29, 34]

Dose by ideal body weight in obese patients [34]

Creatinine Clearance	Dose
>40 ml/min:	25 mg/kg PO Q6H
20–40 ml/min	25 mg/kg PO Q12H
10–19 ml/min	25 mg/kg PO Q24H
<10 ml	25 mg/kg PO Q48H
Hemodialysis	25–50 mg/kg Q48-72H, dose after HD on HD days

Goal peak of 30–80 mg/L to be obtained 2 h post dose after 3–5 days of therapy [34].
Alternative recommendation: peak 50–100 mg/L with trough 25–50 mg/L [29].

Azole Antifungals

Commonly utilized systemic azole antifungal agents used in the neutropenic patient population include fluconazole, voriconazole, posaconazole, and isavuconazonium sulfate. Azole antifungals impair the synthesis of ergosterol, a vital component in the fungal cell membrane which is analogous to cholesterol in the mammalian cell membrane [35]. This is accomplished by inhibition of 14α-sterol demethylase which is a cytochrome p450 (CYP450) enzyme – this also explains why CYP450 based drug interactions are so common with these agents [35].

Fluconazole

Structure of Fluconazole [36]

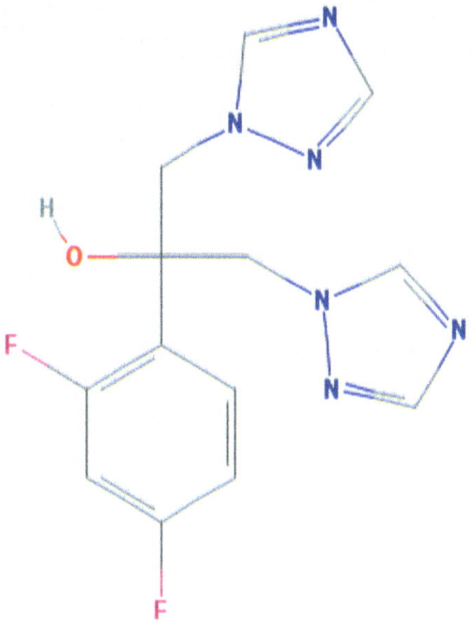

Fluconazole (Diflucan) demonstrates activity against the vast majority of *Candida albicans, Candida keyfr, Candida dublinensis, Candida tropicalis, Candida parapsilosis, Candida guillermondii,* and *Candida lusitaniae* [31]. Fluconazole may demonstrate reduced activity against specific strains of *Candida glabrata* due to their propensity to produce efflux pumps to expel azole antifungals [31]. Depending on the efficacy and density of these efflux pumps, higher doses of fluconazole may be an option [31]. *Candida krusei* is intrinsically resistant to fluconazole [31].

Fluconazole is highly active against *Cryptococcus* allowing for its use for maintenance and secondary prophylaxis in the treatment of cryptococcal meningitis [37]. Fluconazole has also been used first-line for mild to moderate pulmonary cryptococcosis and other single sites of infection in the absence of meningitis or cryptococcemia [37].

Fluconazole is generally well tolerated but patients should be monitored for rare cases of hepatotoxicity [38] and QTc prolongation especially in combination with other QTc prolonging drugs including fluoroquinolones [38].

Fluconazole demonstrates excellent bioavailability and therefore the oral route should be utilized unless the patient is unable to tolerate oral medications, such as severe mucositis, or has an active NPO order [31]. Unlike the other azole antifungal agents, fluconazole is renally eliminated which also allows for achievement of urine concentrations 10–20 times the serum concentration [31]. Fluconazole also has the best distribution of the triazoles into the cerebrospinal fluid (CSF) and vitreous fluid with greater than 70% penetration [31].

Fluconazole is considered a mild to moderate inhibitor of CYP450 3A4, 2C9, and 2C19 [39]. Since fluconazole can be administered over a wide range of dosing, please be aware that higher fluconazole doses can result in more clinically significant drug interactions. Examples of agents with potentially clinically significant fluconazole drug interactions include astemizole, certain benzodiazepines (alprazolam, diazepam, midazolam, triazolam), cisapride, clopidogrel, cyclosporine, fentanyl, ifosfamide, lovastatin, oral hypoglycemics, phenytoin, rifabutin, rifampin, simvastatin, sirolimus, tacrolimus, terfenadine, tyrosine kinase inhibitors, and warfarin [40].

Fluconazole dosing – consider adjusted body weight for dosing in obese patients [40]

Candidemia	Loading Dose	800 mg (12 mg/kg) PO/IV ×1
	Maintenance Dose	400 mg (6 mg/kg) PO/IV Q24H
Central Nervous System/Infective Endocarditis	400 (6 mg/kg) to 800 mg (12 mg/kg) PO/IV Q24H	
Candida glabrata infection (Sensitive dose-dependent, SDD)	800 mg (12 mg/kg) PO/IV Q24H	
Oropharyngeal	100–200 mg PO/IV Q24H	
Antifungal prophylaxis	200–400 mg PO/IV Q24H	
Renal adjustment	CrCl <50 ml/min	Reduce MD by 50%
	Hemodialysis	100% of dose after each HD session

Voriconazole

Structure of Voriconazole [39]

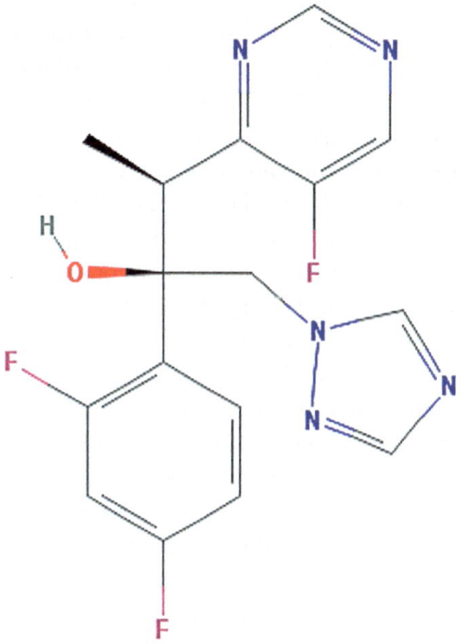

Voriconazole (Vfend) demonstrates similar activity against yeasts compared to fluconazole except that it maintains activity versus *Candida krusei* and may be utilized once susceptibility data has been verified as an oral option for the treatment of fluconazole-resistant, voriconazole-sensitive *Candida glabrata* infections [31]. Voriconazole is FDA approved for the treatment of esophageal candidiasis as well as candidemia and disseminated candidiasis in the skin, abdomen, kidney, bladder wall, and wounds in non-neutropenic patients [31]. Neutropenic patients were excluded from the clinical trial which lead to FDA approval for this indication [41].

Voriconazole has significantly broader antifungal activity than its parent compound fluconazole. Voriconazole is FDA approved for the treatment of invasive aspergillosis and is considered to be the drug of choice for this indication due to lower mortality rates compared to patients randomized to conventional amphotericin B [32]. Voriconazole is also FDA approved for the treatment of invasive fungal infections caused by *Scedosporium apiospermum* and *Fusarium* in patients intolerant of, or refractory to other therapy [41]. *Aspergillus ustus*, which requires amphotericin B therapy, has been reported to cause infections in stem cell transplants receiving voriconazole prophylaxis [42]. In clinical practice, voriconazole is typically considered the drug of choice for *Scedosporium apiospermum* given superior activity compared to amphotericin products [43]. Voriconazole is often used in combination with other potentially active agents such as lipid formulations of amphotericin B or terbinafine for the treatment of Fusariosis in this high risk patient population [8], at least until antifungal susceptibility results are back. Unfortunately voriconazole resistant *Fusarium* is being increasingly reported [8].

Voriconazole lacks activity against mucormycosis and must not be used to treat these life-threatening invasive fungal infections [44].

Voriconazole can cause adverse reactions commonly associated with most of the other azole fungals such as hepatotoxicity, rash, and QTc prolongation [41, 45]. But voriconazole exhibits additional side effects that are more unique. Voriconazole can cause visual disturbances such as blurred vision or color perception issues in up to 30% of patients, typically occurring approximately 30 min after a dose and lasting for up to 30 min – "The Rule of 30" [41, 45]. The site of this usually manageable toxicity is the retina and it has been demonstrated via electroretinography to be reversible following discontinuation [41, 45]. Voriconazole prescribing information recommends that patients not drive when their vision is affected or at night [41]. This needs to be distinguished from central nervous system toxicity (hallucinations and encephalopathy) which occurs in 4.3% of patients [41, 45] and can range from vivid dreams to elaborate visual hallucinations which can be upsetting to patients especially if they are not forewarned about this possibility. Risk for encephalopathy and hallucinations are associated with elevated trough concentrations greater than 5.5 mg/L [45, 46]. Voriconazole is unlike the other azole fungals in that it is a photosensitizer which can result in sunburn-like rashes in 2% of patients and with prolonged utilization, it has been reported to increase the risk of cutaneous squamous cell carcinoma or melanoma [45, 47]. Patients taking voriconazole should limit their exposure to sunlight and use UVA and UVB SPF30+ sunscreen and seek medical attention promptly for new skin lesions. Patients receiving prolonged voriconazole therapy may also experience musculoskeletal pain due to fluorosis and periositis [48]. This has not been associated with other triazole antifungals likely because voriconazole contains 3 fluoride ions per molecule compared to 2 in posaconazole, for example [48].

Voriconazole exhibits excellent bioavailability if separated from meals [41] or enteral feedings [49] by at least 1 h. Voriconazole achieves extensive tissue distribution [41] and achieves clinically significant (>50% penetration) CSF and vitreous concentrations [31]. Voriconazole, unlike fluconazole, does not accumulate in the urine and should not be used for *Candida* urinary tract infections [31].

Voriconazole exhibits substantial variation in hepatic metabolism which inactivates voriconazole primarily via CYP2C19, but also to a lesser extent CYP2C9 and CYP3A4 enzymes [41]. Voriconazole metabolism can demonstrate non-linearity which means that a 50% dose increase can result in a serum concentration increase ranging from 0.4 to 7.7 fold [50].

Genetic polymorphisms in CYP2C19 metabolism appear to represent 30–50% of the inter-patient variability in voriconazole clearance [50]. We are currently evaluating the impact of increasing voriconazole starting dose in rapid CYP2C19 metabolizers and avoiding voriconazole in ultra-rapid CYP2C19 metabolizers [45].

Voriconazole metabolism can be induced by agents such as phenytoin, rifabutin, and rifampin resulting in reduced levels or inhibited by omeprazole resulting in increased levels [41].

Voriconazole is a potent inhibitor of CYP3A4, CYP 2C9, and CYP2C19 which can lead to multiple drug interactions including, but not limited to, the following agents: alprazolam, amlodipine, astemizole, atazanavir, cisapride, clopidogrel, cyclosporine, diazepam, diltiazem, efavirenz, etravirine, felodipine, fentanyl, fosamprenavir, lovastatin, marviroc, midazolam, neviraprine, nifedipine, nisoldipine, omeprazole, oral hypoglycemics, oxycodone, phenytoin, ranolazine, rifabutin,ritonavir, simvastatin, sirolimus, tacrolimus, terfenadine, verapamil, vinblastine, vincristine, and warfarin [45].

Voriconazole dosing – consider adjusted body weight in obese patients [45, 51]		
Invasive Fungal Infections (Aspergillosis, Candidiasis, Fusariosis, Scediosporosis, etc.)	Loading Doses:	6 mg/kg PO/IV BID ×2 doses
	OR 400 mg PO/IV BID ×2 doses	
	Maintenance Doses: 3–4 mg/kg PO/IV BID	
	OR 200 mg to 300 mg PO BID	
Goal trough of 1–5.5 mg/L or random level of 2–6 mg/L to be obtained after 5–7 days [46, 52].		
Renal dysfunction	Renal insufficiency has no effect on voriconazole elimination [41]	

Intravenous voriconazole contains a cyclodextrin solubilizing agent which may accumulate in patients with renal insufficiency [41]. As a result, the prescribing information recommends to avoid intravenous voriconazole in patients with creatinine clearance less than 50 ml/min if possible [41]. This is, however, a theoretical concern and no increase in rates of nephrotoxicity, hepatoxicity, or other adverse effects have been observed in the literature to date despite seven separate retrospective studies [53].

Hepatic dysfunction:	Child-Pugh score-based maintenance dose recommendations are found in the voriconazole prescribing information [41]:
Child Pugh Score A-B:	Reduce voriconazole maintenance dose by 50%
Child Pugh Score C:	Dose reduction required, but no data to guide by how much.

Many neutropenic cancer patients experience acute hepatic dysfunction as a result of their underlying malignancy, cytotoxic chemotherapy, or other medications and Child Pugh score has not been validated in this patient population. Therapeutic drug monitoring can be very helpful in this scenario.

Posaconazole

Structure of Posaconazole [54]

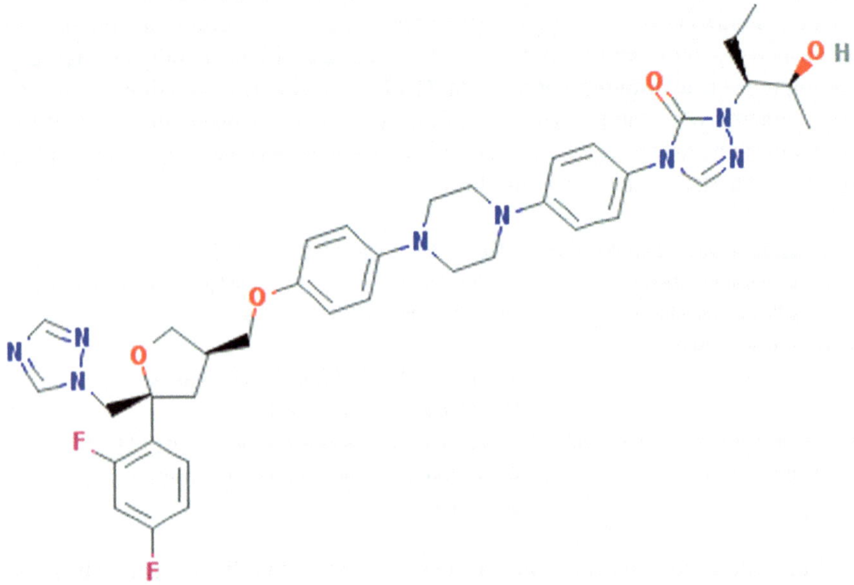

Posaconazole (Noxafil) exhibits a spectrum of activity similar to voriconazole with the notable addition of mucromycosis activity [55]. Posaconazole is FDA approved for prevention and treatment of aspergillosis and candidiasis in high risk patients (MDS/AML receiving induction chemotherapy, allogeneic stem cell transplant recipients with graft-versus-host disease requiring high dose corticosteroids) [56]. Posaconazole has been utilized as salvage therapy for invasive fungal infections, especially against aspergillosis and mucormycosis, but the quantity and quality of this data is limited and based on the use of the original and suboptimal oral liquid formulation [57, 58].

One advantage that posaconazole can claim over voriconazole is tolerability. Posaconazole exhibits an adverse reaction profile comparable to fluconazole therefore patients need only be monitored for hepatotoxicity, QTc prolongation, and rash [59]. Intravenous posaconazole can also cause phlebitis with multiple doses via peripheral vein administration, which is why it is not recommended to give more than one dose prior to central line placement [56].

Posaconazole was originally FDA approved in 2006 only as an oral suspension with 200 mg/5 mL concentration [56]. Posaconazole oral suspension needs to be taken with a meal, ideally a fatty meal, or an enteral feeding such as Boost Plus to increase absorption [56]. Posaconazole is also dependent upon gastric pH to achieve adequate absorption which is why it should not be taken concurrently with proton pump inhibitors and why concurrent acidic ginger ale and/or ascorbic acid can increase absorption [56, 60]. This formulation also exhibits saturable absorption which is why the drug was given as 200 mg/5 mL by mouth 3–4 times per day despite a half-life of greater than 24 h [56–60]. The FDA approval of posaconazole delayed release tablets and an intravenous formulation with a cyclodextrin solubilizing agent eliminated the requirements for low gastric pH and concurrent food intake and thereby greatly improved the pharmacokinetic profile of posaconazole [56].

Posconazole has excellent distribution although its CSF penetration appears to be inferior to fluconazole and voriconazole [55, 56]. Posaconazole is primarily metabolized by UDP-glucoronidation and has no major oxidative, CYP450-mediated metabolites [55, 56]. Posaconazole metabolism can be induced by efavirenz, phenytoin, rifabutin, and rifampin resulting in subtherapeutic concentrations [55, 56]. Posaconazole is a strong inhibitor of CYP450 3A4 specifically and unlike fluconazole and voriconazole does not significantly impact on CYP450 2C9 or 2C19 metabolism [4, 5, 55, 56]. This results in nearly as many drug interactions as voriconazole which include but are not limited to the following: alprazolam, amiodarone, amlodipine, astemizole, cisapride, cyclosporine, diazepam, diltiazem, dofetilide, ergot alkaloids, felodipine, irinotecan, lovastatin, midazolam, maraviroc, nifedipine, nisolidipine, oral hypglycemics, ritonavir, sildenafil, simvastatin, sirolimus, tacrolimus, tadalafil, terfenadine, triazolam, vardenafil, verapamil, vinblastine, and vincristine [55, 56, 59].

Posaconazole dosing [56, 59, 60]

Posaconazole delayed release 100 mg tablets

  Take 3 tablets (300 mg) by mouth twice per day on Day 1

  Do not omit loading doses, required to rapidly achieve therapeutic concentrations

  Then take 3 tablets (300 mg) by mouth daily starting on Day 2

Posconazole intravenous: 300 mg IV Q12H ×2 doses then 300 mg IV Q24H

  To be administered via central line to reduce risk of phlebitis with multiple doses

Posaconazole 200 mg/5 mL oral suspension is inferior from a pharmacokinetic standpoint – **recommend use of newer formulations** if possible.

Prophylaxis:	200 mg/5 mL PO TID with meals or 1 can Boost plus or Ensure plus
Treatment [57, 58]:	200 mg/5 mL PO QID with meals of 1 can Boost plus or Ensure plus 400 mg/10 mL PO BID with meals or 1 can Boost plus or Ensure plus at discharge

Consider use of a "posconazole bundle" [60] to maximum absorption:

  Ascorbic acid 250–500 mg PO with each posaconazole dose in addition to acidic beverage, and heavy snack /meal/nutritional supplement.

  No concurrent proton pump inhibitors.

Renal dysfunction:	No impact on posaconazole clearance [56] Due to potential for cyclodextrin accumulation, the prescribing information discourages use of IV posaconazole in patients with CrCl <50 mL/min [56] – note that is a theoretical concern and based on data with IV voriconazole [53], the risk of increased toxicity in patients with renal impairment is probably minor.
Hepatic dysfunction:	No dose adjustment is recommended [56]

Isavuconazonium Sulfate

Structure of isavuconazonium sulfate [61], pro-drug of isavuconazole

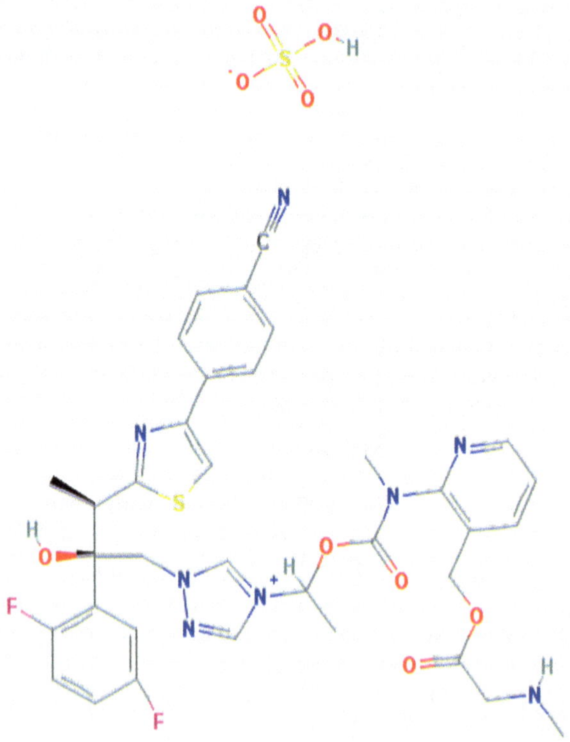

Structure of isavuconazole [62], the active antifungal agent

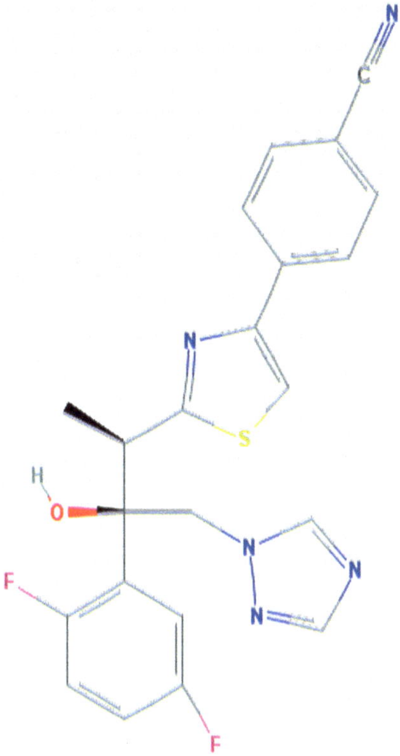

Isavuconazonium sulfate (Cresemba) is a water-soluble pro-drug for isavuconazole (ISV), which exhibits a spectrum of activity very similar to posaconazole [63]. Cresemba was FDA approved for the treatment of invasive aspergillosis and invasive mucormycosis on March 6, 2015 [64]. Phase II clinical trial data is available in the setting of antifungal prophylaxis in neutropenic acute leukemics [65] and treatment of esophageal candidiasis [66].

Cresemba is generally well tolerated and with similar adverse reaction profile to fluconazole or posaconazole [63] and exhibited a slightly lower incidence and severity of ocular toxicity and hepatotoxicity than voriconazole in a randomized trial for aspergillosis [67]. Unlike the other azoles, isavuconazole does not cause QTc prolongation and actually displays a modest QTc shortening effect [63, 64].

Isavuconazonium sulfate is rapidly cleaved to ISV following administration of oral capsules or intravenously, which is why there is no need for a cyclodextrin solubilizing agent [63, 64]. Isavuconazonium sulfate may also be prematurely converted to ISV if the product is shaken or sent via a pneumomatic tube system [63,

64]. Cresemba exhibits excellent oral absorption which is not affected by concurrent oral intake or gastric pH [63, 64]. Isavuconazole displays a large volume of distribution, is highly protein bound, and has a prolonged half-life of greater than 100 h [63]. Given the extremely long half-life, the use of the recommended loading doses is critical – without loading, it can take weeks to reach the therapeutic steady state concentration [63]. Isavuconazole should not be used to treat fungal urinary tract infections due to poor urinary penetration [63]. Data is lacking on central nervous penetration – distribution into the brain parenchyma is likely to be superior to penetration into cerebrospinal fluids [68].

Isavuconazole is primarily metabolized by CYP 3A4 [63]. Concurrent strong CYP 3A4 inducers such as rifampin, carbamazepine, St. John's wort, or barbiturates are contraindicated due to high probability of resulting in subtherapeutic ISV concentrations [63]. Concurrent strong 3A4 inhibitors such as high dose ritonavir (400 mg PO BID) and ketoconazole are not advised due to potential for supratherapeutic ISV concentrations [63].

Isavuconazole is a mild to moderate inhibitor of CYP 3A4 [68] which can be beneficial in patients receiving essential medications that are 3A4 substrates if the only other alternatives would be strong CYP 3A4 inhibitors such as voriconazole and posaconazole. Nonetheless, isavuconazole can result in multiple drug interactions including, but not limited to atorvastatin, buproprion, cyclosporine, digoxin, lopinavir-ritonavir, midazolam, mycophenolate mofetil, sirolimus, and tacrolimus [63].

<u>Isavuconazonium sulfate</u> <u>dosing</u> [[63]]
NOTE: Cresemba (isavuconazonium sulfate) is available in 186 mg capsules or 372 mg vials for IV use.
Isavuconazonium sulfate 372 mg = Isavuconazole 200 mg
Cresemba 186 mg #2 (372 mg) PO Q8H ×2 days (6 doses)
then 186 mg #2 (372 mg) PO Daily
Cresemba 372 mg IVPB Q8H ×2 days (6 doses) then 372 mg IVPB Q24H
In clinical trials, the maintenance dosing started 12–24 h after the last loading dose
Do not omit loading doses, required to achieve therapeutic concentrations in timely manner
Swallow capsules whole – do not chew, crush, dissolve, or open the capsules

Renal dysfunction:	No dose adjustment
Hepatic dysfunction:	No dose adjustment required for Child Pugh Class A and B No recommendation for Child Pugh Class C

Echinocandin Antifungals

Structure of caspofungin acetate [69]

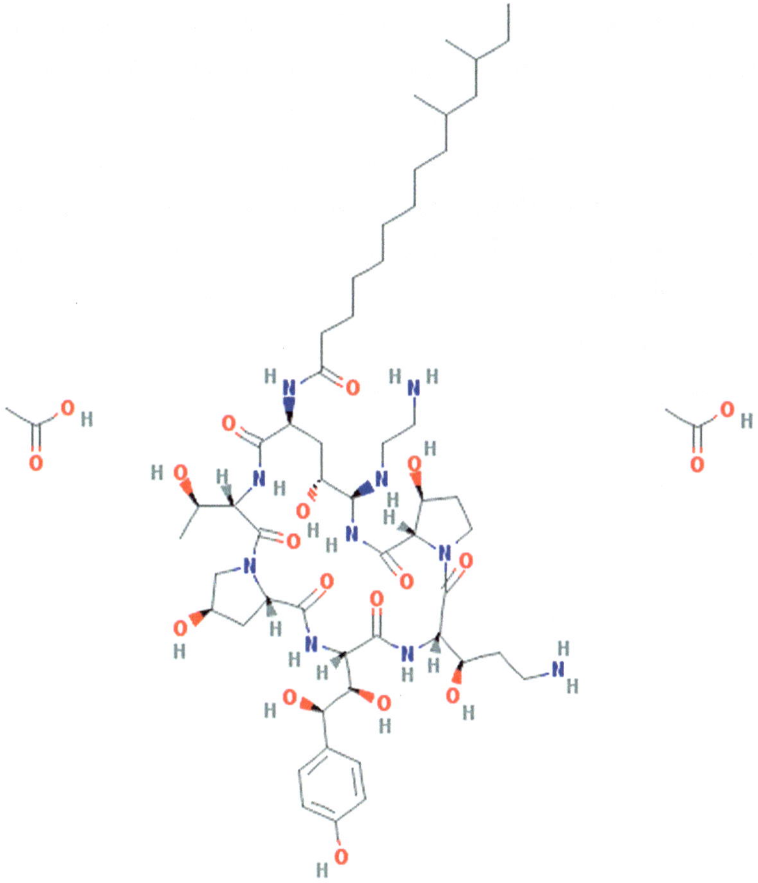

Structure of micafungin [70]

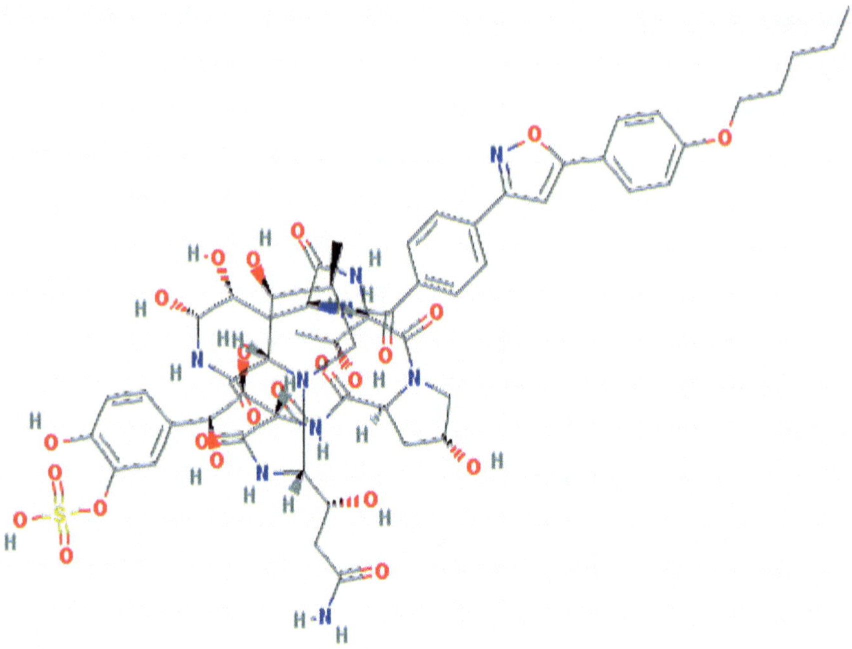

Structure of anidulafungin [71]

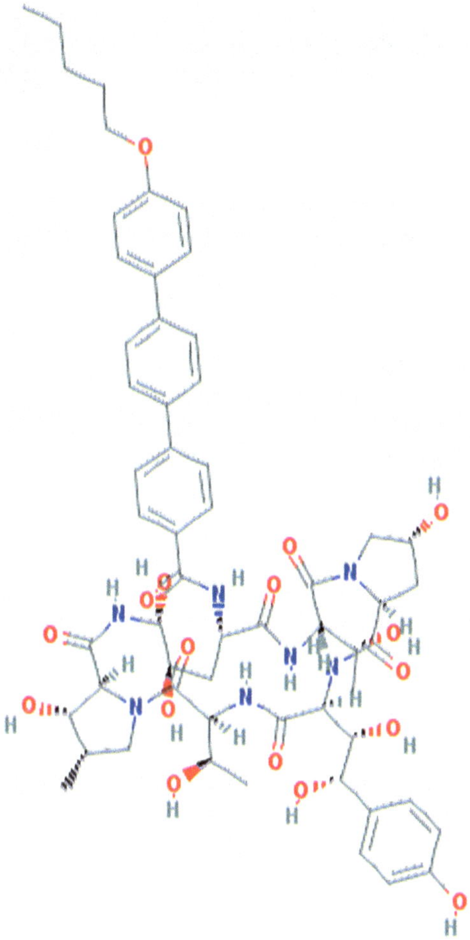

There are currently three FDA approved echinocandin antifungal agents: Caspofungin acetate (Cancidas) approved in 2001 [72], Micafungin (Mycamine) approved in 2005 [73], and Anidulafungin (Eraxis) approved in 2006 [74, 75].

The echinocandin antifungals inhibit the synthesis of β-1,3-D-glucan which is an essential component in the fungal cell wall [72–75]. The excellent tolerability of this antifungal class is likely due in part to the fact that there is no mammalian analogous structure to β-1,3-D-glucan unlike ergosterol and cholesterol in the fungal and mammalian cell membranes that are involved in the mechanisms of action of both amphotericin B and azole antifungals.

The echinocandins all display fungicidal activity against most *Candida* species and are considered to be the initial treatment of choice for candidemia [31, 76]. *Candida parapsilosis* intrinsically exhibits higher echinocandin MICs than other

Candida strains and azole antifungals may be preferred over echinocandins for this species [31]. While echinocandins are typically considered to be the initial treatment of choice for invasive *Candida glabrata* infections [31], the incidence of echinocandin-resistant *Candida glabrata* appears to be on the rise likely due to overuse of these agents [77]. While echinocandins have been proposed as the preferred treatment for *Candida auris*, echinocandin-resistant strains have been reported in addition to those with azole-resistance and/or amphotericin B resistance [7].

Unfortunately, echinocandins only exhibit fungistatic activity against *Aspergillus* [76]. As a result, echinocandin monotherapy is not recommended for the primary treatment of invasive aspergillosis, but only for salvage therapy [32]. Combination therapy of echinocandins with either azole antifungals or amphotericin B formulations have been proposed but are not recommended in the 2016 Aspergillus IDSA guidelines [32]. A randomized clinical trial comparing voriconazole monotherapy to voriconazole and anidulafungin for invasive aspergillosis failed to demonstrate a statistically significant mortality difference between monotherapy and combination therapy [78]. Post-hoc analysis suggested that galactomannan positivity might identify a patient population that could benefit from combination therapy [78]. *Asperillus ustus* infections have been reported to break through echinocandin prophylaxis in stem cell transplant recipients [42].

The echinocandin antifungals as a class are usually very well tolerated [76]. Hepatotoxicity has been reported but appears to be less common than seen with either amphotericin B formulations or voriconazole [79]. Histamine-mediated infusion reactions have been rarely reported [72–75]. Case reports in critically ill patients and animal studies have suggested that the echinocandins may impair left ventricular function in critically ill patients, but further research is needed regarding the incidence and clinically significance of this proposed toxicity [80].

The echinocandin antifungals must be administered intravenously due to insignificant oral bioavailability [72–76]. The echinocandins are all highly protein bound mostly to albumin and distribute well in clinically relevant human tissues with the exception of the central nervous system and urinary tract [31, 72–76]. Caspofungin acetate is either metabolized by hydrolysis or N-acetylation or spontaneously degrades to an inactive open-ring formulation [72]. Caspofungin acetate does require a loading dose of 70 mg to rapidly achieve target concentration [72]. Caspofungin acetate dose reduction to 35 mg/day is recommended in patients with moderate liver dysfunction (Child-Pugh score B) and the prescribing information states that inadequate data exists in patients with severe liver dysfunction (Child-Pugh score C) [72]. Micafungin metabolism is metabolized initially by arylsufatase and is not significantly affected by CYP3A oxidative metabolism [73]. Micafungin does not require a loading dose and also does not require dose modification for patients with mild to severe liver dysfunction (Child-Pugh score A-C) [73]. Anidulafungin is not significantly hepatically metabolized and instead demonstrates slow chemical breakdown under physiological conditions to an inactive, open-ring peptide [75]. Anidulafungin does require a loading dose of twice the maintenance dose but does not require dose modification even in the setting of severe liver dysfunction [75]. None of the echinocandins are significantly affected by renal dysfunction [72–76].

Echinocandin drug interactions vary slightly between agents but are typically less problematic than those encounted with the azole antifungals. Despite the lack of a clinically significant pharmacokinetic drug interaction of caspofungin acetate with cyclosporine or tacrolimus, the combination of caspofungin acetate with cyclosporine has been reported to result in increased risk of transaminitis [72]. A recent publication suggests that the caspofungin acetate-cyclosporine interaction is unlikely to cause increased risk of hepatotoxicity [81]. Caspofungin acetate metabolism may be increased by hepatic cytochrome inducers such as rifampin, nevirapine, efavirenz, carbamazepine, dexamethasone, or phenytoin [72]. Micafungin drug interactions are rarely clinically important – the prescribing information notes that patients receiving concurrent sirolimus, nifedipine, or itraconazole should be monitored for signs of toxicity and reduce the dose of the concurrent agent if necessary [73] although it is in fact rarely necessary. When anidulafungin was first released, the recommended initial diluent contained a high percentage of ethanol which created concerns regarding possible drug interactions with metronidazole or use in patients with either a history of substance abuse or religious prohibitions to ethanol ingestion [74]. This is no longer a problem since the current prescribing information recommends reconstitution with either sterile water, D5W, or normal saline [75]. There are no known clinically relevant drug interactions with anidulafungin [75].

<u>Caspofungin acetate dosing</u> [73]

Caspofungin acetate 70 mg IV ×1 then 50 mg IV Q24H
for all indications except esophageal candidiasis

For esophageal candidiasis:	50 mg IV Q24H without loading dose	
Concurrent CYP inducers:	70 mg IV Q24H	

(rifampin, nevirapine, efavirenz, carbamazepine, dexamethasone, or phenytoin)
Higher doses of caspofungin acetate (100–150 mg IV Q24H) have been utilized and tolerated but without evidence for clinical superiority [82].

Renal dysfunction:	No dose adjustment	
Hepatic dysfunction:	No dose adjustment required for Child Pugh Class A	
	Child Pugh Class B:	Consider 70 mg IV ×1 then 35 mg IV Q24H
	Child Pugh Class C:	Insufficient data

<u>Micafungin dosing</u> [74]

Candidemia, Acute Disseminated Candidiasis, *Candida* Peritonitis and Abscesses	100 mg IV Q24H
Esophageal Candidiasis	150 mg IV Q24H
Prophylaxis of *Candida* Infections in Stem Cell Transplant Recipients	50 mg IV Q24H
Antifungal Prophylaxis – Acute Leukemia or	100 mg IV Q24H [83]

Myelodysplastic Syndrome after Chemotherapy (not FDA approved)	
Renal dysfunction:	No dose adjustment
Hepatic dysfunction:	No dose adjustment
Anidulafungin dosing [76]	
Candidemia and other *Candida* Infections (intra-abdominal, peritonitis)	200 mg IV ×1 then 100 mg IV Q24H
Esophageal Candidiasis	100 mg IV ×1 then 50 mg IV Q24H
Combination therapy for Aspergillosis (not FDA approved)	200 mg IV ×1 then 100 mg IV Q24H [78]
Renal dysfunction:	No dose adjustment
Hepatic dysfunction:	No dose adjustment
Hepatic dysfunction:	No dose adjustment required for Child Pugh Class A and B No recommendation for Child Pugh Class C

Summary Table

Antifungal	Notes
Amphotericin B	Broad fungicidal activity
	Resistance most common in *Candida lusitaniae, Aspergillus terreus, Scedosporium* species, and *Trichosporin beigelii.* Also reports of resistant *Candida auris* and *Fusarium* species
Amphotericin B deoxycholate (Fungizone)	"Amphoterrible"
	Tolerability limited by infusion reactions, nephrotoxicity, and potassium and magnesium wasting.
	Premedication with hydrocortisone 50 mg PO/IV, acetaminophen 650 mg PO, and/or diphenhydramine 25–50 mg PO/IV may reduce infusion reactions. Rigors can be treated with opioids such as hydromorphone 0.5 mg IV.
	While NS 500 mL IV before and after each dose may reduce or delay nephrotoxicity, use of lipid formulations are safer from renal standpoint.
	Extended infusion amphotericin B deoxycholate reported to cause fewer infusion reactions and nephrotoxicity.
	Monitor patient closely for hypokalemia and hypomagnesemia. Consider scheduled oral potassium and/or magnesium supplementation. Amiloride 5–10 mg PO BID may also be utilized to reduce amphotericin associated hypokalemia.
Amphotericin B Colloidal Dispersion (ABCD) or Amphotericin B Cholesteryl Sulfate (Amphotec)	Less nephrotoxic than amphotericin B deoxycholate
	Highest incidence of infusion rates of all amphotericin formulations.

(continued)

Antifungal	Notes
Amphotericin B Lipid Complex (ABLC, Abelcet)	Less nephrotoxic than amphotericin B deoxycholate
	Infusion reactions comparable to amphotericin B deoxycholate
Liposomal Amphotericin B (Ambisome)	Lowest incidence of infusion reactions and nephrotoxicity of the amphotericin formulations
	Can rarely cause acute, severe atypical infusion reactions which may require change to an alternative agent
Nystatin (Mucostatin)	Comparable *in vitro* activity to amphotericin B but utilized clinically almost exclusively for oral, cutaneous, and vaginal candidiasis.
	Intravenous liposomal nystatin may have a role in the future for the treatment of invasive fungal infections in neutropenic patients, but remains an investigational agent at this time.
Flucytosine (Ancobon)	Active against *Candida* except *Candida krusei*, *Cryptococcus*, and *Aspergillus*
	Used almost exclusively for treatment of Cryptococcal meningitis in combination with amphotericin B
	Dose limiting toxicity is myelosuppression
	Therapeutic drug monitoring has been proposed but long turn-around time prevents from this from being clinically useful given usual 2 week duration of therapy
Fluconazole (Diflucan)	Active against *Candida albicans, Candida keyfr, Candida dublinensis, Candida tropicalis, Candida parapsilosis, Candida guillermondii, and Candida lusitaniae*. Reduced activity against *Candida glabrata* due to efflux pump production – high dose fluconazole may be effective against sensitive dose-dependent *Candida glabrata*
	Active against *Cryptococcus* – used for maintenance therapy and secondary prophylaxis in the treatment of cryptococcal meningitis or first line for mild to moderate cryptococcosis
	Usually well tolerated but may cause hepatotoxicity, QTc prolongation, and rash
	Excellent bioavailability, can be used oral or IV at same dosing
	Best azole penetration into urinary tract, central nervous system, and the eye
	Mild to moderate inhibitor of CYP450 3A4, 2C9, and 2C19

(continued)

Antifungal	Notes
Voriconazole (Vfend)	Activity against yeasts comparable to fluconazole but also usually active against *Candida krusei* and may be active against fluconazole resistant *Candida glabrata*. First line treatment of invasive aspergillosis (except for *Aspergillus ustus*) and scedosporiosis. Increasing reports of resistant *Fusarium* in clinical isolates. Not active against mucormycosis.
	Monitor patients for hepatotoxicity, QTc prolongation, rash, visual disturbances, and encephalopathy including hallucinations
	Photosensitizer – avoid prolonged sunlight exposure, cover up, and use high quality sunscreens of SPF30+
	Long term use can result in fluorosis and periostitis
	Excellent bioavailability if taken at least 1 h from food or enteral feedings.
	Excellent distribution including clinically significant central nervous system and ocular penetration. Not recommended for urinary tract infections.
	Metabolized primarily by CYP2C19 with substantial generic variance in metabolism
	CYP2C19 genotyping may prove to be useful in determine initial voriconazole dose
	Therapeutic drug monitoring is recommended especially in the treatment setting
	Potent inhibitor of CYP 3A4, CYP2C9, and CYP2C19 leading to many clinically relevant drug interactions
Posaconazole (Noxafil)	Activity comparable to voriconazole except for addition of activity against mucormycosis
	FDA approved for antifungal prophylaxis, not treatment other than for esophageal candidiasis
	Tolerability comparable to fluconazole but monitor for hepatoxicity, QTc prolongation, and rash
	Available in delayed release tablets and intravenous formulations which achieve more reliable concentrations than the original oral suspension formulation which requires concurrent food intake as well as acidic gastric environment for optimal absorption
	Potent inhibitor of CYP 3A4 resulting in many clinically relevant drug interactions

(continued)

Antifungal	Notes
Isavuconazonium sulfate (Cresemba)	Activity comparable to posaconazole
	FDA approved for treatment of aspergillosis and mucormycosis
	Tolerability comparable to fluconazole and posaconazole, monitor for hepatotoxicity and rash
	Does not cause QTc prolongation, modest QTc shortening effect
	Excellent bioavailability, available in capsules or IV formulation
	Prolonged half-life, loading dose during first 2 days of therapy is essential otherwise sub-therapeutic for weeks
	Distributes well into body tissues except urinary tract
	Data lacking on central nervous system penetration but better brain parenchyma penetration than into cerebrospinal fluid
	Primarily metabolized by CYP 3A4 – avoid concurrent potent inhibitors or inducers of CYP 3A4
	Mild to moderate inhibitor of CYP 3A4 which may result in less significant drug interactions than voriconazole or posaconazole
Echinocandins Caspofungin acetate (Cancidas) Micafungin(Mycamine) Anidulafungin (Eraxis)	Fungicidal against most *Candida* species, first line for Candidemia
	Less potent against *Candida parapsilosis*
	Case reports of echinocandin resistance in *Candida glabrata* and *Candida auris*
	Fungistatic against *Aspergillus* other than *Aspergillus ustus*, which is resistant to echinocandins
	Have been used in combination with amphotericin or azole antifungals for salvage therapy of aspergillosis but randomized clinical trial failed to demonstrate mortality benefit except perhaps in galactomannan assay positive cases
	Usually very well tolerated, monitor for hepatotoxicity
	Rare histaminic infusion related reactions
	May impair left ventricular ejection fraction in critically ill patients
	Limited to intravenous administration
	Excellent distribution except for central nervous system and urinary tract
	Caspofungin acetate and anidulafungin require loading dose on day 1 of therapy, but micafungin does not
	Consider caspofungin acetate dose reduction in patients with moderate liver dysfunction, not required for micafungin or anidulafungin
	Caspofungin acetate requires dose increase if given with enzyme inducers
	Caspofungin acetate-cyclosporine drug interaction may result in increased incidence of transaminitis
	Micafungin drug interactions with sirolimus, nifedipine, or itraconazole are rarely clinically significant
	Anidulafungin has no known drug interactions

References

1. National Center for Biotechnology Information. PubChem Compound Database; CID=71311649. https://pubchem.ncbi.nlm.nih.gov/compound/71311649. Accessed 20 Apr 2018.
2. Saravolatz LD, Ostrosky-Zeichner LO, Marr KA, Rex JH, Cohen SH. Amphotericin B: time for a new "Gold Standard". Clin Infect Dis. 2003;37(3):415–25.
3. Amphotericin B deoxycholate prescribing information. X-Gen Pharmaceuticals, Inc. Big Flats, New York. Revised December 2009.
4. Ellis D. Amphotericin B: spectrum and resistance. J Antimicrob Chemother. 2002;49(Suppl 1):7–10.
5. Van Der Linden JWM, Warris A, Verweij PE. Aspergillus species intrinsically resistant to antifungal agents. Med Mycol. 2011;49(Suppl 1):S82–9.
6. Walsh TJ, Melcher GP, Rinaldi MG, Lecciones J, McGough DA, et al. Trichosporin beigelii, an emerging pathogen resistant to amphotericin B. J Clin Microbiol. 1990;28(7):1616–22.
7. Sarma S, Upadhyay S. Current perspective on emergence, diagnosis, and drug resistance in Candida auris. Infect Drug Resist. 2017;10:155–65.
8. Stempel JM, Hammond SP, Sutton DA, Weiser LM, Marty FM. Invasive fusariosis in the voriconazole era: single center 13-year experience. Open Forum Infect Dis. 2015;2(3):ofv099. https://doi.org/10.1093/ofid/ofv099. eCollection 2015 Sep
9. Patel R. Antifungal agents. Part 1. Amphotericin B preparation and flucytosine. Mayo Clinical Proceedings. 1998;73(12):1205–25.
10. Eriksson U, Seifert B, Schaffner A. Comparsion of effects of amphotericin B deoxycholate infused over 4 or 24 hours. Br Med J. 2010;322:1–6.
11. Karimzadeh I, Farsaei S, Khalili H, Dashti-Khavidak S. Are salt loading and prolonging infusion period effective in prevention of amphotericin B induced nephrotoxicity? Expert Opin Drug Safety. 2012;11(6):969–83.
12. Bearden T, Muncey LA. The effect of amiloride on amphotericin B-induced hypokalemia. J Antimicrob Chemother. 2001;48:109–11.
13. Hamill RJ. Amphotericin B formulations: a comparative review of efficacy and toxicity. Drugs. 2013;73(9):919–34.
14. Wingard JR, White MH, Anaissie E, Raffalli JR, Goodman J, et al. A randomized, double-blind comparative trial evaluating the safety of liposomal amphotericin B versus amphotericin B lipid complex in the empirical treatment of febrile neutropenia. Clin Infect Dis. 2000;31:1155–63.
15. Bowden R, Chandrasekar P, White MH, Pietrelli L, Gurwith M, et al. A double-blind, randomized, controlled trial of amphotericin B colloidal dispersion verus amphotericin B for treatment of invasive aspergillosis in immunocompromised patients. Clin Infect Dis. 2002;35(4):359–66.
16. Roden MM, Nelson LD, Knudsen TA, Jarosinski PF, Starling JM, et al. Triad of acute infusion-related reactions associated with Liposomal Amphotericin B. Clin Infect Dis. 2003;36:1213–20.
17. Pham P, Bartlett JG. Amphotericin B. Johns Hopkins ABX Guide. Accessed 4–20-18.
18. Cornely OA, Maertens J, Bresnik M, Ebrahimi R, Ullmann AJ, et al. Liposomal amphotericin B as initial therapy for invasive mold infections: a randomized trial comparing a high-loading dose regimen with standard dosing (AmBiLoad trial). Clin Infect Dis. 2007;44:1289–97.
19. Gubbins PO, Amsden JR, McConnell SA, Anaissie EJ. Pharmacokinetics and Buccal Mucosal Concetrations of 15 mg/kg total dose of liposomal amphotericin B as single dose, weekly dose, or daily dose in peripheral stem cell transplant patients. Antimicrob Agents Chemother. 2009;53(9):3664–74.
20. Cordonnier C, Mohty M, Faucher C, Pautas C, Robin M, et al. Safety of weekly high dose of liposomal amphotericin B for prophylaxis of invasive fungal infection in immunocompromised patients. Int J Antimicrob Agents. 2008;31:135–41.

21. Annino L, Chierichini A, Anaclerico B, Finolezzi E, Norata M, et al. Prospective phase II single-center study of the safety of a single very high dose of liposomal amphotericin B for antifungal prophylaxis in patients with acute myeloid leukemia. Antimicrob Agents Chemother. 2013;57(6):2596–602.
22. Rijinders BJ, Cornelissen JJ, Slobbe L, Becker MJ, Doorduign JK, et al. Aerosolized liposomal amphotericin B for the prevention of invasive pulmonary aspergillosis during prolonged neutropenia. Clin Infect Dis. 2008;46:1401–11.
23. National Center for Biotechnology Information. PubChem Compound Database; CID= 6433272. https://pubchem.ncbi.nlm.nih.gov/compound/6433272. Accessed 27 Aug 2018.
24. Ng AW, Wasan KM, Lopez-Berestein G. Development of liposomal polyene antibiotics: an historical perspective. J Pharm Pharm Sci. 2003;6(1):67–83.
25. Offner F, Krcmery V, Boogaerts M, Doyen C, Engelhard D, et al. Liposomal nystatin in patients with invasive aspergillosis refractory to or intolerant of amphotericin B. Antimicrob Agents Chemother. 2004;48(12):4808–12.
26. Pam PA, Bartlett JG. Nystatin. Johns Hopkins ABX Guide. Accessed 8-27-18.
27. National Center for Biotechnology Information. PubChem Compound Database; CID=3366. https://pubchem.ncbi.nlm.nih.gov/compound/3366. Accessed 24 Apr 2018.
28. Ancobon (flucytosine) capsules prescribing information. Valeant Pharmaceuticals International. Costa Mesa, California. Revised May 2006.
29. Vermes A, Guchelaar H-J, Dankert J. Flucytosine: a review of its pharmacology, clinical indications, pharmacokinetics, toxicity, and drug interactions. J Antimicrob Chemother. 2000;46(2):171–9.
30. Day JN, Chau TTH, Wolbers M, Mai PP, Dung NT, et al. Combination antifungal therapy for cryptococcal meningitis. N Engl J Med. 2013;14:1291–302.
31. Pappas PG, Kauffman CA, Andes DR, Clancy CJ, Marr K, et al. Clinical practice guideline for the management of candidiasis: 2016 update by the Infectious Diseases Society of America. Clin Infect Dis. 2016;62(4):e1–e50.
32. Patterson TG, Thompson GR, Denning DW, Fishman JA, Hadley S, Herbrectht R, et al. Practice guidelines for the diagnosis and management of aspergillus: 2016 update. Clin Infect Dis 2–16. 63(4):e1–e60.
33. Merry M, Boulware DR. Cryptococcal meningitis treatment strategies affected by the explosive cost of fluctyosine in the United States: a cost-effectiveness analysis. Clin Infect Dis. 2016;62(12):1564–8.
34. Pham P, Bartlett JG. Flucytosine. Johns Hopkins ABX Guide. Accessed 4-24-18.
35. Ghannoum MA, Rice LB. Antifungal agents: mode of action, mechanisms of resistance, and correlation of these mechanisms with bacterial resistance. Clin Microbiol Rev. 1999;12(4):501–17.
36. National Center for Biotechnology Information. PubChem Compound Database; CID=3365. https://pubchem.ncbi.nlm.nih.gov/compound/3365. Accessed 24 Apr 2018.
37. Perfect JR, Dismukes WE, Dromer F, Goldman DL, Graybill JR, et al. Clinical practice guidelines for the management of cryptococcal disease: 2010 update by the Infectious Diseases Society of America. Clin Infect Dis. 2010;50:291–322.
38. Zeuli JD, Wilson JW, Estes LL. Effect of combined fluroquinolone and azole use on QT prolongation in hematology patients 2013; 57(3): 1121–1127.
39. National Center for Biotechnology Information. PubChem Compound Database; CID=71616. https://pubchem.ncbi.nlm.nih.gov/compound/71616. Accessed 24 Apr 2018.
40. Pham P, Bartlett JG. Fluconazole. Johns Hopkins ABX Guide. Accessed 4-24-18.
41. Vfend (Voriconazole) prescribing information. Roerig, division of Pfizer. New York. Revised June 2010.
42. Pavie J, Lacroix C, Hermoso DG, Robin M, Ferry C, et al. Breakthrough disseminated aspergillus ustus infection in allogeneic hematopoietic stem cell transplant reccipients receiving voriconazole or caspofungin prophylaxis. J Clin Microbiol. 2005;43(9):4902–4.

43. Goldman C, Akiyama MJ, Torres J, Louie E, Meehan SA. Scedosporium aposperium and role of combination antifungal therapy and GM-CSF. Med Mycol Case Rep. 2016;11:40–3.
44. Lewis RE, Liao G, Wang W, Prince RA, Kontoyiannis DP. Voriconazole pre-exposure selects for breakthrough mucormycosis in a mixed model of Aspergillus fumigatus-Rhizopus oryzae pulmonary infection. Virulence. 2011;2(4):348–55.
45. Pham PA. Bartlett JG. Voriconazole. Johns Hopkins ABX Guide. Accessed 4-29-18.
46. Pascual A, Calandra T, Bolay S, Buclin T, Bille J, Marchetti O. Voriconazole therapeutic drug monitoring in patient with invasive mycoses improves efficacy and safety outcomes. Clin Infect Dis. 2008;46:201–11.
47. Drinkwater DC, Davidson-Moncada J, Heckendorn E, Myers J, Whitman TJ. A patient with ulcerated nodules on his face. Clin Infect Dis. 2014;58:901–2.
48. Thompson GR, Bays D, Cohen SH, Pappagianis D. Fluroride excess in coccidioidomycosis patients receiving long term antifungal therapy. Antimicrob Agents Chemother. 2012;56(1):563–4.
49. Williams D. The effect of enteral nutrition supplements on serum voriconazole levels. J Oncol Pharm Pract. 2011;18(1):128–31.
50. Obeng O, Egelund EF, Asiltan A, Peloquin CA, Johnson JA. CYP2C19 polymorphisms and therapeutic drug monitoring of voriconazole.
51. Dickmeyer NJ, Kiel PJ. Dosing voriconazole in an obese patient. Clin Infect Dis. 2011;53:745.
52. Smith J, Safdar N, Knansinski V, Simmons W, Bhavnani SM, Ambrose PG, Andes D. Antimicrob Agents Chemother. 2006;50:1570–22.
53. Turner RB, Martello JL, Malhorta A. Worsening renal function in patients with baseline renal impairment treated with intravenous voriconazole. Int J Antimicrob Agents. 2015;46(4):362–6.
54. National Center for Biotechnology Information. PubChem Compound Database; CID=468595. https://pubchem.ncbi.nlm.nih.gov/compound/468595. Accessed 29 Apr 2018.
55. Nagappan V, Deresinski S. Posaconazole: A broad-spectrum triazole antifungal agent. Clin Infect Dis. 2007;45:1610–6.
56. Noxafil (posaconazole) prescribing information. Merck. Whitehouse Station. Revised 2014.
57. Walish TJ, Raad I, Patterson TF, Chandrasekar P, Donowitz GR, et al. Treatment in invasive aspergillosis with posaconazole in patients who are refractory to or intolerant of conventional therapy. Clin Infect Dis. 2007;44:2–12.
58. Greenberg RN, Mullane K, van Burik J-AH, Raad I, Abzug MJ, et al. Posconazole as salvage therapy for zygomycosis. Antimicrob Agents Chemother. 2006;50(1):126–33.
59. Pam PA, Bartlett JG. Posconazole. Johns Hopkins ABX Guide. Accessed 4-29-18.
60. Green MR, Woolery JE. Optimising absorption of posaconazole. Mycoses. 2011;54:e775–9.
61. National Center for Biotechnology Information. PubChem Compound Database; CID=72196309. https://pubchem.ncbi.nlm.nih.gov/compound/72196309. Accessed 3 May 2018.
62. National Center for Biotechnology Information. PubChem Compound Database; CID=6918485. https://pubchem.ncbi.nlm.nih.gov/compound/6918485. Accessed 3 May 2018.
63. Miceli MH, Kauffman CA. Isavuconazole: a new broad-spectrum triazole antifungal agent. Clin Infect Dis. 2015;61(10):1558–65.
64. Cresemba (isavuconazonium sulfate) prescribing information. Astellas Pharma Inc. Northbrook. Revised June 2015.
65. Cornely OA, Bohme A, Schmitt-Hoffman A, Ulmann AJ. Safety and pharmacokinetics of isavuconazole as antifungal prophylaxis in acute myeloid leukemia patients with neutropenia. Antimicrob Agents Chemother. 2015;59:2078–85.
66. Viljoen J, Schmitt-Hoffman A, Ghannoum M. A phase 2, randomized, double-blind, multicenter trial to evaluate the safety and efficacy of three dosing regimens of isavuconazole compared to fluconazole in patients with uncomplicated esophageal candidiasis. Antimicro Agents Chemother. 2015;59(3):1671–9.
67. Maertens JA, Raad II, Marr KA, Patterson TF, Kontoyiannis DP, et al. Isavuconazole versus voriconazole for primary treatment of invasive mould disease caused by Aspergillus and

other filamentous fungi (SECURE). Lancet. 2016;387(10020):760–9. https://doi.org/10.1016/S0140-6736(15)01159-9.. Epub 2015 Dec 10
68. Pettit NN, Carver PL. Isavuconazole: a new option for the management of invasive fungal infections. Ann Pharmacother. 2015;49(7):825–42.
69. National Center for Biotechnology Information. PubChem Compound Database; CID=66577041. https://pubchem.ncbi.nlm.nih.gov/compound/66577041. Accessed 3 May 2018.
70. National Center for Biotechnology Information. PubChem Compound Database; CID=477468. https://pubchem.ncbi.nlm.nih.gov/compound/477468. Accessed 3 May 2018.
71. National Center for Biotechnology Information. PubChem Compound Database; CID=166548. https://pubchem.ncbi.nlm.nih.gov/compound/166548. Accessed 3 May 2018.
72. Cancidas (caspofungin acetate) prescribing information. Merck and Company, Inc. Whitehouse Station. Revised Mar 2018.
73. Mycamine (micafungin) prescribing information. Astellas Pharma US, Inc. Northbrook. Revised Aug 2016.
74. Eraxis (anidulafungin) prescribing information. Pfizer. New York. Original prescribing information on February 16, 2006.
75. Eraxis (anidulafungin) prescribing information. Pfizer. New York. Revised January 2018.
76. Chen SC, Slavin MA, Sorrell TC. Echinocandin antifungal drugs in fungal infections: a comparison. Drugs. 2011;17(1):11–41.
77. Perlin DS. Echinocandin resistance in Candida. Clin Infect Dis. 2015;61(Suppl 6):S612–7.
78. Marr KA, Sclamm HT, Herbrect R, Rottinghaus ST, Bow EJ, et al. Combination antifungal therapy for invasive aspergillosis: a randomized trial. Ann Intern Med. 2016;162(2):81–9.
79. Wang J-L, Chang C-H, Young-Xu Y, Chan KA. Systematic review and meta-analysis of the tolerability and hepatotoxicity of antifungals in empirical and definitive therapy for invasive fungal infection. Antimicrob Agents Chemother. 2018;62:2409–19.
80. Koch C, Uhle F, Wolff M, Arens C, Schulte A, Li L, et al. Cardiac effects of echinocandins after central venous administration in adult rats. Antimicrob Agents Chemother. 2018;62(5):1612–9.
81. Nishimoto M, Koh H, Tokuwame A, Makuuchi Y, Kuono M, et al. Drug interactions and safety profiles with concomitant use of casofungin and calcineurin inhibitors in allogeneic haemtolopoietic cell transplantation. Br J Clin Pharmacol. 2017;83(9):2000–7.
82. Betts RF, Nucci M, Talwar D, Gareca M, Queiroz-Telles T, et al. A multi-center double-blind trial of high-dose caspofungin treatment regimen versus standard caspofungin treatment regimen for adjust patients with invasive candidiasis. Clin Infect Dis. 2009;48:1676–84.
83. Epstein DJ, Seo SK, Huang YT, Park JH, Klimek VM, et al. Micafungin versus posaconazole prophylaxis in acute leukemia or myelodysplastic syndrome: a randomized study. J Infect 2018; pii: S0163-4453(18)30132-4. doi: https://doi.org/10.1016/j.jinf.2018.03.015. [Epub ahead of print].

Antimicrobial Prophylaxis

Yanina Pasikhova

Abstract During the period of neutropenia (ANC < 500 cells/mm^3) following cytotoxic chemotherapy and hematopoietic stem cell transplantation (HSCT) oncology patients are at a significant risk for infections (Freifeld et al., Clin Infect Dis 52(4):e56–e93, 2011). Patients with profound neutropenia, defined as ANC < 100 cells/mm^3 are at greatest risk with bacteremia rates reported as high as 20%, often with septic shock and multi-system organ failure (Freifeld et al., Clin Infect Dis 52(4):e56–e93, 2011; Horton et al., Curr Hematol Malig Rep13:59, 2018).

A number of modalities have been evaluated to mitigate the risk of infections in vulnerable oncology patients with neutropenia. Among the most widely utilized has been the use of antimicrobial prophylaxis during the time of afebrile neutropenia. Recommendations for prophylaxis vary based on overall risk of infections as determined by disease state and treatment received. Low risk patients are typically those with solid tumors receiving standard chemotherapy with anticipated neutropenia less than 7 days (Freifeld et al., Clin Infect Dis 52(4):e56–e93, 2011; National Comprehensive Cancer Network. Prevention and treatment of cancer-related infections (Version 1.2018). https://www.nccn.org/professionals/physician_gls/pdf/infections.pdf. Accessed 11 Apr 2018). Such patients do not routinely require bacterial, fungal or viral prophylaxis (Freifeld et al., Clin Infect Dis 52(4):e56–e93, 2011; National Comprehensive Cancer Network. Prevention and treatment of cancer-related infections (Version 1.2018). https://www.nccn.org/professionals/physician_gls/pdf/infections.pdf. Accessed 11 Apr 2018). On the other hand patients undergoing HSCT or those receiving treatment for acute leukemia are considered high risk for infections and thus typically received bacterial, fungal and viral prophylaxis (Freifeld et al., Clin Infect Dis 52(4):e56–e93, 2011; National Comprehensive Cancer Network. Prevention and treatment of cancer-related infections (Version 1.2018). https://www.nccn.org/professionals/physician_gls/pdf/infections.pdf. Accessed 11 Apr 2018).

Y. Pasikhova, PharmD (✉)
Department of Pharmacy, Mofitt Cancer Center, Tampa, FL, USA
e-mail: yanina.pasikhova@moffitt.org

A. P. Velez et al. (eds.), *Infections in Neutropenic Cancer Patients*,
https://doi.org/10.1007/978-3-030-21859-1_10

Keywords Antibacterial prophylaxis · Antifungal Prophylaxis · Antiviral prophylaxis · Prophylactic antibiotics · Neutropenia · Allogeneic HSCT · Autologous HSCT · Induction chemotherapy · Gastrointestinal mucositis

Antibacterial Prophylaxis

Patients with profound neutropenia, defined as ANC < 100 cells/mm^3 are at the greatest infectious risk, with bacteremia rates reported as high as 20%, often with septic shock and multi-system organ failure [1, 2]. Numerous studies, some as early as the 1980's, have demonstrated that the use of prophylactic antibiotics during the period of neutropenia can decrease febrile episodes and documented infections [1]. However, more recent meta-analyses have demonstrated risk reduction in all-cause and infection-related mortality in high risk patients receiving fluoroquinolone prophylaxis compared to placebo [4, 5].

.As a result a number of guidelines including those from American Society for Blood and Marrow Transplantation (ASBMT), Infectious Disease Society of America (IDSA), the National Comprehensive Cancer Network (NCCN), and European Society for Blood and Marrow Transplantation (EBMT) endorse this practice in high risk oncology patients with hematologic malignancies undergoing both induction chemotherapy and HCST [1, 3, 6, 7]. Emergence of resistance to fluoroquinolones, concern for superinfections with *Clostridium difficile* and alteration in the microbiome have brought this practice to question.

Who [1, 3, 6, 7]

High risk patients

- Anticipated prolonged profound neutropenia (ANC $\leq$ 100 cells/mm^3 for >7 days)
- Anticipated prolonged neutropenia (ANC $\leq$ 500 cells/mm^3 for >10 days)
- Allogeneic HSCT
- Acute leukemia
  - Induction
  - Consolidation/maintenance

What [1, 3, 8]

- Fluoroquinolone
  - Ciprofloxacin 500 mg PO/IV BID

  - Levofloxacin 500 mg PO/IV Daily
    - Preferred when additional viridans group streptococcal coverage indicated
- Oral third generation cephalosporin
  - Patients not able to receive a fluoroquinolone (i.e. intolerance, drug interactions, resistance)

When [1, 3, 6, 7]

- Start of neutropenia
  - Some protocols will start at time of chemotherapy
- Continue until resolution of neutropenia

Antifungal Prophylaxis

Neutropenic oncology patients are at risk of fungal infections, both from yeast and mold. Similar to antibacterial prophylaxis, primary antifungal prophylaxis will be guided by patient's risk for developing such infections. Patients with solid tumors and anticipated neutropenia duration of less than 7 days are considered low risk for fungal infections and routinely do not receive antifungal prophylaxis [3]. Widespread use of antifungal prophylaxis with fluconazole has been linked to increasing rates of infections with fluconazole resistant yeasts and therefore is only recommended in oncology patients with invasive *Candida* infection rates of 6–10% [1]. Patients who fall into this category are those with acute leukemia and oral or gastrointestinal mucositis secondary to chemotherapy, pre-engraftment allogeneic HSCT recipients and autologous HSCT recipients with mucositis [1, 3].

Similar to anti-*Candida* prophylaxis, the need for prophylaxis against Aspergillus varies according to patient's disease and chemotherapy used for treatment of the disease [1]. In general patients with a baseline risk of greater than 6% for invasive aspergillosis appear to benefit from primary prophylaxis with a mold active agent [1]. This includes patients with acute myeloid leukemia (AML) receiving induction chemotherapy and patients with advanced myelodysplastic syndromes (MDS) undergoing intensive treatment [1, 3]. In allogeneic HSCT recipients prophylaxis with a mold active agent should be considered in patients with graft-versus-host disease (GVHD) on high dose steroids($\geq$1 mg per kg prednisone equivalent) with or without anti-thymocyte globulin (ATG) or TNF blockade (infliximab), anticipated prolonged neutropenia of 2 weeks or greater or those with longstanding neutropenia immediately prior to HSCT [1, 3, 7, 9]. For details on specific agents and secondary antifungal prophylaxis please refer to chapter on antifungals and invasive fungal infections.

Pneumocystis jiroveci (PCP) is a life-threatening fungal infection that affects immunocompromised oncology and non-oncology patients. Patients with hematologic malignancies and those undergoing a HSCT are at greatest risk [3, 10]. Prophylaxis has been recommended in patients with baseline risk of PCP greater than or equal to 6.2%, with a number needed to treat is 19 to prevent a singe case of PCP [11]. This includes patients with acute lymphoblastic leukemia (ALL), allogeneic HSCT recipients, patients receiving alemtuzumab, corticosteroids (≥20 mg per day prednisone or equivalent for ≥4 weeks), purine analog therapy (fludarabine) and temozolomide in combination with radiation therapy [3, 7, 10].

Who [1, 3, 7, 9, 10]

- Yeast
  - Acute leukemia
  - Allogeneic HSCT
    - Pre-engraftment phase
  - Autologous HSCT recipients with mucositis
    - Pre-engraftment phase
- Mold
  - AML
    - Induction
  - Allogeneic HSCT
    - Graft-versus-host disease (GVHD)
      - On high doses of steroids (≥1 mg per kg prednisone equivalent)
    - Anticipated prolonged neutropenia of 2 weeks or greater
    - Longstanding neutropenia immediately prior to HSCT
- PCP
  - ALL
  - Alemtuzumab
  - Allogeneic HSCT recipients
  - Corticosteroids (≥20 mg per day prednisone or equivalent for ≥4 weeks)
  - Purine analog therapy (fludarabine)
  - Temozolomide + radiation therapy

What [1, 3, 7, 10, 12]

- Yeast
  - Fluconazole 200–400 mg PO/IV Daily
  - Micafungin 50–100 mg IV Daily
  - Amphotericin B products
- Mold
  - Posaconazole suspension 200 mg PO TID
  - Posaconazole tablets 300 mg PO/IV BID x 1 day then daily
  - Voriconazole 200 mg PO/IV BID
  - Amphotericin B products
  - Isavuconazonium
- PCP
  - First-line: Trimethoprim/ sulfamethoxazole 1 SS (80/400 mg) PO Daily or 1 DS (160/800 mg) PO TIW
  - Second-line: dapsone, atovaquone, pentamidine aerosol or intravenous

When [1, 3, 7, 10]

- Yeast and mold
  - Start of neutropenia
  - Continue until resolution of neutropenia
    - In patients with GVHD, until resolution of GVHD
- PCP
  - ALL
    - Throughout anti-leukemic therapy
  - Alemtuzumab
    - Minimum of 2 months after drug discontinuation and until CD4 ≥ 200 cells/moL
  - Allogeneic HSCT recipients
    - At least 6 months and while on immunosuppression
  - Corticosteroids (≥20 mg per day prednisone or equivalent for ≥4 weeks)
    - At least while on therapy

- Purine analog therapy (fludarabine)
  - Until CD4 ≥ 200 cells/moL
- Temozolomide + radiation therapy
  - At least while on therapy

Antiviral Prophylaxis (Herpes Viruses)

Herpes viruses are large encapsulated deoxyribose nucleic acid (DNA) viruses that can cause acute primary infections and then persist within the host in non-infectious form [13]. Under appropriate conditions herpes viruses have the ability to reactivate and cause latent infections, which may be clinically very different than the primary infection [13]. There are eight types of human herpes virus, and all have been implicated to some extent in human disease. The purpose of this section is to review prophylaxis in neutropenic oncology patients against three of the human herpes viruses; herpes simplex virus 1 (HSV-1), herpes simplex virus 2 (HSV-2) and varicella zoster virus (VZV) [13].

.Similar to antibacterial prophylaxis, antiviral prophylaxis against HSV 1/2 and VZV is only warranted in high risk, seropositive neutropenic oncology patients [1, 3]. However, risk factors other than neutropenia have been linked to reactivation of HSV and VZV, thus even in absence of neutropenia patients receiving therapy with proteasome inhibitors, alemtuzumab, corticosteroids for GVHD and purine analog therapy should receive prophylaxis [1, 3].

Who [1, 3]

- Acute leukemia (seropositive for HSV or VZV or history of chicken pox)
- Alemtuzumab
- Allogeneic HSCT (seropositive donor or recipient for HSV or VZV)
- Allogeneic HSCT with GVHD receiving corticosteroids
- Autologous HSCT (seropositive for HSV or VZV)
- Proteasome inhibitors (bortezomib, carfilzomib, ixazomib)
- Purine analog therapy (fludarabine)

What [3]

- Acyclovir 400–800 mg PO BID
- Famciclovir 250 mg PO BID
- Valaciclovir 500 mg PO BID-TID

When [1, 3]

- Acute leukemia
  - HSV
    - Continue until resolution of neutropenia or mucositis, whichever occurs later
- Alemtuzumab
  - HSV
    - Minimum of 2 months after drug discontinuation and until CD4 $\geq$ 200 cells/moL
- Allogeneic HSCT
  - HSV
    - Continue until resolution of neutropenia or mucositis, whichever occurs later
  - VZV
    - For at least 1 year after HSCT
- Autologous HSCT
  - HSV
    - Continue until resolution of neutropenia or mucositis, whichever occurs later
  - VZV
    - 6–12 months after HSCT
- Proteasome inhibitors (bortezomib, carfilzomib, ixazomib)
  - VZV
    - During active therapy
- Purine analog therapy (fludarabine)
  - HSV and VZV
    - During active therapy or longer depending on degree of immunosuppression

Key Points

	Who	What	When
Antibacterial	Anticipated prolonged profound neutropenia (ANC ≤ 100 cells/mm3 for >7 days) Anticipated prolonged neutropenia (ANC ≤ 500 cells/mm3 for >10 days) Allogeneic HSCT Acute leukemia Induction Consolidation/maintenance	Fluoroquinolone Ciprofloxacin 500 mg PO/IV BID Levofloxacin 500 mg PO/IV Daily (Preferred when additional viridans group streptococcal coverage indicated) Oral third generation cephalosporin Patients not able to receive a fluoroquinolone (i.e. intolerance, drug interactions, resistance)	Start of neutropenia Some protocols will start at time of chemotherapy Continue until resolution of neutropenia
Antifungal: yeast	Acute leukemia Allogeneic HSCT Pre-engraftment phase Autologous HSCT recipients with mucositis Pre-engraftment phase	Fluconazole 200–400 mg PO/IV Daily Micafungin 50–100 mg IV Daily Amphotericin B products	Start of neutropenia Continue until resolution of neutropenia

(continued)

	Who	What	When
Antifungal: mold	AML Induction Allogeneic HSCT Graft-versus-host disease (GVHD) Anticipated prolonged neutropenia of 2 weeks or greater Longstanding neutropenia immediately prior to HSCT	Posaconazole suspension 200 mg PO TID Posaconazole tablets 300 mg PO/IV BID x 1 day then daily Voriconazole 200 mg PO/IV BID Amphotericin B products Isavuconazonium	Start of neutropenia Continue until resolution of neutropenia In patients with GVHD, until resolution of GVHD
Antifungal: PCP	ALL Alemtuzumab Allogeneic HSCT recipients Corticosteroids (≥20 mg per day prednisone or equivalent for ≥4 weeks) Purine analog therapy (fludarabine) Temozolomide + radiation therapy	First line Trimethoprim/sulfamethoxazole 1 SS (80/400 mg) PO Daily or 1 DS (160/800 mg) PO TIW Second-line Dapsone, atovaquone, pentamidine aerosol or intravenous	ALL Throughout anti-leukemic therapy Alemtuzumab Minimum of 2 months after drug discontinuation and until CD4 ≥ 200 cells/moL Allogeneic HSCT recipients At least 6 months and while on immunosuppression Corticosteroids (≥20 mg per day prednisone or equivalent for ≥4 weeks) At least while on therapy Purine analog therapy (fludarabine) Until CD4 ≥200 cells/moL Temozolomide + radiation therapy At least while on therapy

(continued)

	Who	What	When
Antiviral	Acute leukemia (seropositive for HSV or VZV or history of chicken pox) Alemtuzumab Allogeneic HSCT (seropositive donor or recipient for HSV or VZV) Allogeneic HSCT with GVHD receiving corticosteroids Autologous HSCT (seropositive for HSV or VZV) Proteasome inhibitors (bortezomib, carfilzomib, ixazomib) Purine analog therapy (fludarabine)	Acyclovir 400–800 mg PO BID Famciclovir 250 mg PO BID Valaciclovir 500 mg PO BID-TID	Acute leukemia HSV (Continue until resolution of neutropenia or mucositis, whichever occurs later) Alemtuzumab HSV (Minimum of 2 months after drug discontinuation and until CD4 ≥ 200 cells/moL) Allogeneic HSCT HSV (Continue until resolution of neutropenia or mucositis, whichever occurs later) VZV (For at least 1 year after HSCT) Autologous HSCT HSV (Continue until resolution of neutropenia or mucositis, whichever occurs later) VZV (6–12 months after HSCT) Proteasome inhibitors (bortezomib, carfilzomib, ixazomib) VZV (During active therapy) Purine analog therapy (fludarabine) HSV and VZV (During active therapy or longer depending on degree of immunosuppression)

References

1. Freifeld AG, Bow EJ, Sepkowitz KA, Boeckh MJ, Ito JI, Mullen CA, Raad II, Rolston KV, Young J-AH, Wingard JR. Clinical practice guideline for the use of antimicrobial agents in Neutropenic patients with cancer: 2010 update by the Infectious Diseases Society of America. Clin Infect Dis. 2011;52(4):e56–93. https://doi.org/10.1093/cid/cir073.
2. Horton LE, Haste NM, Taplitz RA. Curr Hematol Malig Rep. 2018;13:59.. https://doi.org/10.1007/s11899-018-0435-0
3. National Comprehensive Cancer Network. Prevention and treatment of cancer-related infections (Version 1.2018). https://www.nccn.org/professionals/physician_gls/pdf/infections.pdf. Accessed 11 Apr 2018.
4. Leibovici L, Paul M, Cullen M, Bucaneve G, Gafter-Gvili A, Fraser A, Kern WV. Antibiotic prophylaxis in neutropenic patients. Cancer. 2006;107:1743–51. https://doi.org/10.1002/cncr.22205.

5. Gafter-Gvili A, Fraser A, Paul M, Vidal L, Lawrie TA, van de Wetering MD, Kremer LCM, Leibovici L. Antibiotic prophylaxis for bacterial infections in afebrile neutropenic patients following chemotherapy. Cochrane Database Syst Rev. 2012;(1):CD004386. https://doi.org/10.1002/14651858.CD004386.pub3.
6. Tomblyn M, Chiller T, Einsele H, Gress R, Sepkowitz K, Storek J, et al. Guidelines for preventing infectious complications among hematopoietic cell transplantation recipients: a global perspective. Biol Blood Marrow Transplant. 2009;15(10):1143–238. https://doi.org/10.1016/j.bbmt.2009.06.019.
7. Ullmann AJ, Schmidt-Hieber M, Bertz H, Heinz WJ, Kiehl M, Kruger W, et al. Infectious diseases in allogeneic haematopoietic stem cell transplantation: prevention and prophylaxis strategy guidelines 2016. Ann Hematol. 2016;95:1435–55. https://doi.org/10.1007/s00277-016-2711-1. Updated version of the Infectious Diseases Workng Group of the German Society for Hematology and Medical Oncology guideline
8. Yemm KE, Barreto JN, Mara KC, Dierkhising RA, Gangat N, Tosh PK. A comparison of levofloxacin and oral third-generation cephalosporins as antibacterial prophylaxis in acute leukaemia patients during chemotherapy-induced neutropenia. J Antimicrob Chemother. 2018;73(1):204–11. https://doi.org/10.1093/jac/dkx338.
9. Kontoyiannis DP. Antifungal prophylaxis in hematopoietic stem cell transplant recipients: the unfinished tale of imperfect success. Bone Marrow Transplant. 2011;46(2):165–73. https://doi.org/10.1038/bmt.2010.256. Epub 2010 Nov 1.
10. Johan Maertens, on behalf of the 5th European Conference on Infections in Leukaemia (ECIL-5), a joint venture of the European Group for Blood and Marrow Transplantation (EBMT), the European Organisation for Research and Treatment of Cancer (EORTC), the Immunocompromised Host Society (ICHS) and the European LeukemiaNet (ELN), Simone Cesaro, on behalf of the 5th European Conference on Infections in Leukaemia (ECIL-5), a joint venture of the European Group for Blood and Marrow Transplantation (EBMT), the European Organisation for Research and Treatment of Cancer (EORTC), the Immunocompromised Host Society (ICHS) and the European LeukemiaNet (ELN), Georg Maschmeyer, on behalf of the 5th European Conference on Infections in Leukaemia (ECIL-5), a joint venture of the European Group for Blood and Marrow Transplantation (EBMT), the European Organisation for Research and Treatment of Cancer (EORTC), the Immunocompromised Host Society (ICHS) and the European LeukemiaNet (ELN), Hermann Einsele, on behalf of the 5th European Conference on Infections in Leukaemia (ECIL-5), a joint venture of the European Group for Blood and Marrow Transplantation (EBMT), the European Organisation for Research and Treatment of Cancer (EORTC), the Immunocompromised Host Society (ICHS) and the European LeukemiaNet (ELN), J. Peter Donnelly, on behalf of the 5th European Conference on Infections in Leukaemia (ECIL-5), a joint venture of the European Group for Blood and Marrow Transplantation (EBMT), the European Organisation for Research and Treatment of Cancer (EORTC), the Immunocompromised Host Society (ICHS) and the European LeukemiaNet (ELN), Alexandre Alanio, on behalf of the 5th European Conference on Infections in Leukaemia (ECIL-5), a joint venture of the European Group for Blood and Marrow Transplantation (EBMT), the European Organisation for Research and Treatment of Cancer (EORTC), the Immunocompromised Host Society (ICHS) and the European LeukemiaNet (ELN), Philippe M. Hauser, on behalf of the 5th European Conference on Infections in Leukaemia (ECIL-5), a joint venture of the European Group for Blood and Marrow Transplantation (EBMT), the European Organisation for Research and Treatment of Cancer (EORTC), the Immunocompromised Host Society (ICHS) and the European LeukemiaNet (ELN), Katrien Lagrou, on behalf of the 5th European Conference on Infections in Leukaemia (ECIL-5), a joint venture of the European Group for Blood and Marrow Transplantation (EBMT), the European Organisation for Research and Treatment of Cancer (EORTC), the Immunocompromised Host Society (ICHS) and the European LeukemiaNet (ELN), Willem J. G. Melchers, on behalf of the 5th European Conference on Infections in Leukaemia (ECIL-5), a joint venture of the European Group for Blood and Marrow Transplantation

(EBMT), the European Organisation for Research and Treatment of Cancer (EORTC), the Immunocompromised Host Society (ICHS) and the European LeukemiaNet (ELN), Jannik Helweg-Larsen, on behalf of the 5th European Conference on Infections in Leukaemia (ECIL-5), a joint venture of the European Group for Blood and Marrow Transplantation (EBMT), the European Organisation for Research and Treatment of Cancer (EORTC), the Immunocompromised Host Society (ICHS) and the European LeukemiaNet (ELN), Olga Matos, on behalf of the 5th European Conference on Infections in Leukaemia (ECIL-5), a joint venture of the European Group for Blood and Marrow Transplantation (EBMT), the European Organisation for Research and Treatment of Cancer (EORTC), the Immunocompromised Host Society (ICHS) and the European LeukemiaNet (ELN), Stéphane Bretagne, on behalf of the 5th European Conference on Infections in Leukaemia (ECIL-5), a joint venture of the European Group for Blood and Marrow Transplantation (EBMT), the European Organisation for Research and Treatment of Cancer (EORTC), the Immunocompromised Host Society (ICHS) and the European LeukemiaNet (ELN), Catherine Cordonnier, on behalf of the 5th European Conference on Infections in Leukaemia (ECIL-5), a joint venture of the European Group for Blood and Marrow Transplantation (EBMT), the European Organisation for Research and Treatment of Cancer (EORTC), the Immunocompromised Host Society (ICHS) and the European LeukemiaNet (ELN), on behalf of the 5th European Conference on Infections in Leukaemia (ECIL-5), a joint venture of the European Group for Blood and Marrow Transplantation (EBMT), the European Organisation for Research and Treatment of Cancer (EORTC), the Immunocompromised Host Society (ICHS) and the European LeukemiaNet (ELN), Samir Agrawal, Murat Akova, Alexandre Alanio, Mahmoud Aljurf, Dina Averbuch, Thomas Berg, Ola Blennow, Stéphane Bretagne, Roger Brüggemann, Thierry Calandra, Elio Castagnola, Simone Cesaro, Catherine Cordonnier, Oliver Cornely, Rafael De La Camara, Peter Donnelly, Lubos Drgona, Rafael Duarte, Hermann Einsele, Dan Engelhard, Corrado Girmenia, Ruth Hargreaves, Philippe Hauser, Jannick Helweg-Larsen, Raoul Herbrecht, Hans Hirsch, Petr Hubacek, Christopher Kibbler, Galina Klyasova, Michal Kouba, Bart-Jan Kullberg, Katrien Lagrou, Per Ljungman, Johan Maertens, Vincent Mallet, Oscar Marchetti, Georg Maschmeyer, Olga Matos, Willem Melchers, Malgorzata Mikulska, Patricia Munoz, Christina Orasch, Livio Pagano, Antonio Pagliuca, Olaf Penack, George Pettrikos, Zdenek Racil, Patricia Ribaud, Valérie Rizzi-Puechal, Emmanuel Roilides, Janos Sinko, Anna Skiada, Monica Slavin, Jan Styczynski, Frederic Tissot, Lorraine Tweddle, Florian van Boemmel, Marie von Lilienfeld-Toal, Claudio Viscoli, Katherine Ward, Craig Wood; ECIL guidelines for preventing Pneumocystis jirovecii pneumonia in patients with haematological malignancies and stem cell transplant recipients, J Antimicrob Chemother, 71 9, 2016, 2397–2404, https://doi.org/10.1093/jac/dkw157.

11. Stern A, Green H, Paul M, Vidal L, Leibovici L. Prophylaxis for Pneumocystis pneumonia (PCP) in non-HIV immunocompromised patients. Cochrane Database Syst Rev. 2014;(10):CD005590. https://doi.org/10.1002/14651858.CD005590.pub3.
12. Mellinghoff SC, Panse J, Alakel N, et al. Ann Hematol. 2018;97:197. https://doi.org/10.1007/s00277-017-3196-2.
13. Rao KB. Herpes viruses – an overview. J Pharm. 2014;4(10):39–41.

Antimicrobial Stewardship in Immunocompromised Hosts

Wonhee So

Abstract Although an antimicrobial stewardship program (ASP) as a primary tool to combat global development of antimicrobial resistance has been widely accepted in the last decade, the key principles of ASP have not always been adopted in patients with significant immune defects. Multiple barriers exist for implementing ASP in this population: physician's perceptions regarding the immunocompromised as sicker patients and fear of poor outcomes, a wide range of possible infectious etiologies with diagnostic uncertainty, complexity in making early diagnosis, impaired inflammatory responses, and difficulty in controlling the source of infections due to thrombocytopenia, and limited surgical interventions. However, ASP in the immunocompromised hosts is an important patient safety measure as development of multidrug-resistant (MDR) pathogens is an emerging problem. This chapter discusses strategies and the need for ASP in the immunocompromised host with cancer.

Keywords Antimicrobial stewardship program (ASP) · Formulary Management · Drug Interactions · Early de-escalation in febrile neutropenic patients · Antimicrobial Restriction · Prospective audit and feedback · Microbiological data · Duration of therapy · Antifungal stewardship · Biomarkers · Rapid Diagnostics · Intravenous to oral

Goals and Opportunities of ASP in Immunocompromised Hosts

ASP aims to optimize clinical outcomes while minimizing unintended consequences of antimicrobial use such as toxicity, collateral damage and development of resistance as well as to reduce cost without compromising outcome [1]. The same goals apply to the patients with immune deficiency. Furthermore, opportunities for

W. So (✉)
San Antonio, TX, USA

A. P. Velez et al. (eds.), *Infections in Neutropenic Cancer Patients*,
https://doi.org/10.1007/978-3-030-21859-1_11

ASP exist for both prophylaxis and treatment in the immunocompromised host by optimizing drug selection, dose, route and duration.

ASP Modalities in Immunocompromised Hosts

Formulary Management

ASP plays a crucial role in formulary decisions of antimicrobials. Formulary choices must balance the accessibility of key treatment options for immunocompromised hosts and adverse effects including drug costs. For example, ASP streamlines the hospital formulary based on potential drug interactions between antimicrobials and chemotherapy/immunosuppressants (e.g., nafcillin-tacrolimus interaction via CYP3A4 v. no interaction between oxacillin-tacrolimus for treatment of methicillin-susceptible *Staphylococcus aureus* (MSSA) infections), cost (e.g. cost effectiveness analysis between ceftaroline and other anti-methicillin-resistant *S. aureus* (MRSA) agents) and spectrum of coverage (e.g., limitation of the use of ceftolozane/tazobactam or ceftazidime/avibactam v. a narrower spectrum agent when broad spectrum coverage is not necessary). ASP should also assess drug supply and usage (e.g., drug shortages in cefepime, piperacillin-tazobactam), changes in price (e.g., increase in price of flucytosine, IV erythromycin), and availability of newer agents with similar usage (e.g., isavuconazole v. posaconazole) to modify hospital-wide guidelines without compromising patient care. Once a drug is added to the formulary, ASP provides oversights on the implementation of restricted use via staff education, ordering requirements in the computer software program, and preauthorization (antimicrobial restriction) and prospective audit and feedback.

Antimicrobial Prophylaxis During Neutropenia

While there are guidelines available for antimicrobial prophylaxis in cancer patients including a recent review of biologicals and targeted therapies [2], collaboration between infectious diseases specialists and hematologists is essential to risk stratify who would need antimicrobial prophylaxis and to formulate the prophylaxis regimen due to complex immune dysfunctions in these hosts and unique infectious risks associated with certain stage of diseases or chemotherapeutic agents. For example, a review of infectious complications of patients who received blinatumomab, an anti-CD19 immunotherapy for relapsed/refractory B-cell acute lymphoblastic leukemia (ALL), noted a high rate (15%) of nodular, possible mold pneumonia [3]. While NCCN guidelines recommend fluconazole or micafungin as an antifungal prophylaxis for most ALL patients [4], more potent anti-mold prophylaxis was advocated when blinatumomab recipients presented with baseline neutropenia (i.e. ANC < 500 cells/μL) due to relapsed or refractory disease.

Fluoroquinolone prophylaxis has been recommended by the guidelines for high-risk patients who are going to be profoundly neutropenic for >7 days [4]. Despite the rising concern over fluoroquinolone resistance, a recent Cochrane review confirmed the reduction in mortality and infection rates still outweighs the risk of resistance, costs and adverse events associated with fluoroquinolone prophylaxis [5]. In the meantime, there are studies showing different classes of antibiotics such as third-generation cephalosporins or sulfamethoxazole-trimethoprim provided similar outcomes as fluoroquinolone prophylaxis [5, 6]. ASP should play a role in antimicrobial prophylaxis by closely monitoring local patterns of resistance, recommending alterative prophylaxis if needed based on prior infectious history or other clinical characteristics, and recommending antibacterial prophylaxis only in selected high-risk patients, but not in all neutropenic patients.

Choice of Agents for Neutropenic Fever

While many clinicians prefer IV antibiotics in the setting of neutropenic fever, oral antibiotics such as a combination of fluoroquinolone (i.e., ciprofloxacin or levofloxacin) plus amoxicillin/clavulanate (or clindamycin for those with a penicillin allergy) have been recommended for outpatient empirical therapy [7]. Adherence to the guidelines and adoption of the established tools for risk assessment provide ASP opportunities. There are several tools such as MASCC (Multinational Association for Supportive Care in Cancer) scoring and clinical criteria that may be used to differentiate who can be treated as an outpatient versus inpatient. The joint guideline by ASCO (American Society of Clinical Oncology) and IDSA (Infectious Diseases Society of America) endorses the use of a more recently validated tool, CISNE (the Clinical Index of Stable Febrile Neutropenia) score, which is more sensitive and specific in solid tumors for this purpose [7].

Regarding the inpatient management of neutropenic fever, IDSA guidelines recommend a variety of anti-pseudomonal beta-lactam antibiotics in the absence of complications (e.g., hypotension, pneumonia, and colonization of resistant organisms) [8]. While comparative studies did not find differences in clinical or safety outcomes amongst various agents either as monotherapy or in combination [9], institutions can streamline their preferred agents for febrile neutropenia from an ASP perspective. Colonization with resistant organisms poses a substantial risk for infection and a high mortality in immunocompromised hosts [10]. ASP should prescreen patients at highest risk for infections with MDR organisms to tailor individualized empiric antibiotic recommendations. For example, empiric use of carbapenems should be advocated if there is a history of MDR *Pseudomonas* aeruginosa or extended-spectrum β-lactamase (ESBL) producing *Enterobacteriaceae*. Otherwise, it should be reserved when narrower spectrum anti-pseudomonal agents can be utilized.

Also, ASP should limit antibiotics with Gram-positive coverage such as MRSA in accordance with current guidelines. For example, vancomycin is not recommended as initial empiric therapy for neutropenic fever in the absence of a catheter-related infection, skin or soft-tissue infection, pneumonia or hemodynamic instability [8]. The use of empiric antibiotics with anti- vancomycin-resistant *Enterococcus* (VRE) activity once febrile neutropenia develops for those with VRE colonization is under debate. Recent studies showed no difference in mortality between the empiric linezolid group and the control group [11] and no impact on mortality from delayed VRE bloodstream infection treatment [12].

Early De-escalation After Neutropenic Fever

IDSA guidelines for neutropenic fever published in 2011 recommend the initial regimen be continued until clear signs of marrow recovery (i.e., an increasing absolute neutrophils count (ANC) that exceeds 500 cells/μL) in patients with unexplained fever [8]. There have been several recent studies that evaluated early de-escalation of antibiotics. Le Clech *et al* compared the outcomes of early antibiotic de-escalation in two phases for patients with hematologic malignancy with fever of unknown origin (FUO) [13]; in the first phase all antibiotics were stopped 48 h after resolution of fever as recommended by the ECIL-4 guidelines [14], and in the second phase antibiotics were stopped on day 5 whether febrile or afebrile. The composite endpoint defined as in-hospital mortality, intensive care unit (ICU) admission, relapse of febrile neutropenia ≤48 h after discontinuation of antibiotics in afebrile patients or a new documented infection in patients with persistent fever were not different between the two groups and the duration of antibiotics was shorter in the second group (7 v. 5 days, p = 0.002). While having limitations inherent to a nonrandomized trial, such as, a longer duration of neutropenia in the first group (20 v. 12 days, p = 0.01) and different types of chemotherapy and stem cell transplant between the groups, the study demonstrated the feasibility of early de-escalation in febrile neutropenic patients with a hematologic malignancy. In another study by Aguilar-Guisado *et al*, early de-escalation of antibiotics after 72 h of apyrexia and clinical recovery irrespective of neutrophil count recovery was evaluated [15]. This was a superiority, open-label, randomized, controlled phase 4 trial from six hospitals in Spain which included 156 high-risk febrile neutropenic patients with hematological malignancies but without microbiologically or clinically documented infection. When compared to the control group (i.e., anti-pseudomonal antibiotics were continued until ANC > 500 cells/μL), the experimental group showed significantly shorter days of empirical antimicrobials (16.1 v. 13.6 days, p = 0.026) with similar rates of adverse events. One out of 78 and three out of 79 patients died from the experimental and control group, respectively.

Two recent studies specifically assessed early de-escalation in hematopoietic stem cell transplantation recipients (HSCT). The first study by Snyder *et al* compared the rates of recurrent fever, *Clostridium difficile*-associated infection, length of stay, intensive care unit (ICU) admission, in-hospital mortality, need for re-escalation of therapy, rate of positive blood cultures and pharmacoeconomic impact between the early de-escalation group (i.e., empiric antibiotics were de-escalated to prophylaxis after 5 days if defervesced) and control group [16]. They found no difference in the rate of recurrent fever (15% in early de-escalation group v. 19% in control group, 90% CI, −0.088 to 0.163) and in other clinical outcomes, but showed a significant decrease in antimicrobial use in the early de-escalation group which resulted in an estimated antimicrobial cost reduction per 1000 transplant days of approximately $10,000 ($22,300 v. $32,760, p = 0.012).

The second study in HSCT patients by Gustinetti *et al* is a single center study from Italy and compared clinical and economical outcomes between early de-escalation (i.e., de-escalation to a narrower spectrum β-lactam or switching to fluoroquinolone prophylaxis or discontinuation within 96 h in afebrile patients) and late de-escalation (i.e., de-escalation after 96 h) [17]. Failure of de-escalation/discontinuation was defined as escalating or restarting antibiotic therapy, having a blood stream infection or fever recurrence within 96 h from de-escalation/discontinuation. In the early de-escalation group (n = 26), the failure of de-escalation occurred in 4 patients (15.4%, 4/26) including a fever recurrence (n = 1), bartholinitis (n = 1), and bacteremia (n = 2). Of note, these bacteremias were not recurrences of previous infections and all failures were successfully treated with escalation of antibiotic therapy. In the late de-escalation group, the failure of de-escalation occurred in 6 patients (19%, 6/31) which included 2 bacteremia (one *Pseudomonas putida*, and one *Enterococcus faecium*) and fever recurrence. None of these cases resulted in septic shock or death. In multivariate analyses, the presence of blood stream infection was associated with early de-escalation, which reflects their antimicrobial de-escalation practice driven by microbiologic culture regardless of count recovery.

In summary, early de-escalation and discontinuation of broad spectrum antipseudomonal antibiotics in febrile neutropenic patients is feasible while the timing for early de-escalation varies amongst studies. Until newer international guidelines address these aforementioned studies, ASP should be mindful of these results and may consider early de-escalation in selected patients in consultation with infectious diseases clinicians and the hematologist/oncologist.

Clinical Pathway

The 2016 Infectious Diseases Society of America (IDSA) guideline for implementing an ASP endorses the use of facility-specific clinical practice guidelines [18]. Studies have shown that an interdisciplinary development of such guidelines improved awareness and uptake of clinical pathways via multifaceted dissemination and an implementation strategy [18]. Highly employed clinical guidelines for cancer, HSCT and solid organ transplant patients included febrile neutropenia, antifungal prophylaxis, treatment of invasive fungal infections and cytomegalovirus prophylaxis [19]. An institutional antimicrobial use clinical pathway should be based on consensus guidelines, local susceptibility data and cost [9]. For example,

Metan *et al* replaced a carbapenem with piperacillin/tazobactam ± amikacin as a first-line empiric antibacterial regimen except in high risk patients after experiencing a high incidence of carbapenem-resistant Gram-negative bacilli in patients with neutropenic fever [20]. High risk patients were defined as known colonizers with ESBL-producing Enterobacteriaceae who presented with severe sepsis, septic shock, nosocomial pneumonia, or recently transferred from the ICU with a high prevalence of MDR Gram-negative bacilli. This led to a significant reduction in carbapenem use without affecting mortality.

Antimicrobial Restriction

Not only restricting certain antimicrobials that require infectious diseases consultation or an indication for use when prescribing, but also optimizing the duration of antimicrobial use is an important ASP strategy. For example, a simple reminder of daily carbapenem use to prescribers or an automatic email to reassess the duration of certain targeted broad spectrum antibiotics can be used to limit the duration.

Prospective Audit and Feedback

If resources and manpower are available, a prospective audit and feedback (PAF) based on a review of empiric therapy, de-escalation or escalation based on clinical and microbiological data, and duration of therapy should be implemented by the ASP. PAF can be very labor intensive, and identification of appropriate patients for intervention can be challenging if not supported by a computerized surveillance system. The key is allocation of necessary resources, a persistent effort by dedicated, well-trained personnel, and ongoing communication with clinicians [18].

Antifungal Stewardship

While many ASPs have focused initial efforts on reducing inappropriate antibiotic use in awareness of the perils of resistant bacteria, antifungal stewardship should be in place given the evidence of poor use of antifungals which has showed low adherence to guidelines or labeling [21–24] and emergence of resistant organisms, namely azole-resistant *Aspergillus fumigatus* [25], echinocandin-resistant *Candida glabrata* [26], and MDR *Candida auris* [27]. Similar to antibacterial prophylaxis, antifungal prophylaxis is recommended for high-risk patients but not for low-risk patients with anticipated neutropenia less than 7 days. Institutions caring for large numbers of high-risk patients should have local guidelines for antifungal prophylaxis directed against *Candida, Aspergillus, Mucormycosis, Pneumocystis jiroveci* and a surveillance program for early diagnosis of invasive fungal infections. For example, use of early chest CT [28] or quantitative polymerase chain reaction (PCR) assays targeting *Rhizomucor, Lichtheimia, Mucor/Rhizopus* has been advocated for early diagnosis of mucormycosis [29]. The *Aspergillus* galactomannan (GM) test is relatively specific for *Aspergillus*, but β-1,3-D-glucan (BDG) is a component of the cell wall of most fungi and thus has low specificity. Due to the reduced sensitivities and specificities of BDG or *Aspergillus* GM tests, use of these tests are limited and results should be interpreted in conjunction with other clinical, microbiological and radiological findings. For example, the sensitivity of the *Aspergillus* GM test decreases if a patient has already been on an antifungal; a persistently positive GM is associated with higher mortality; and persistent BDG can occur despite resolution of fungal infection [30]. As more biomarkers become available, the ASP should evaluate if each test alone or in combination is valuable in antifungal stewardship and if so, then develop a pathway utilizing these tools for de-escalation or early escalation of antifungals.

Use of Biomarkers

Procalcitonin has been extensively studied as an ASP tool, but its role in neutropenic patients is less clear. For example, complicating factors of routine post-transplant physiology and the effect of transplant-specific therapies such as anti-thymocyte globulin caused an elevated procalcitonin level which was not associated with infection [31]. Despite concerns about potentially limited procalcitonin production in neutropenic patients, a review of 30 articles on the use of procalcitonin in this population concluded procalcitonin may be able to discriminate fever due to systemic infections from non-infectious etiologies [32]. Based on the reported procalcitonin levels in febrile neutropenic patients, the authors reported that values less than 0.5 ng/mL are less likely to occur in patients with infection and a delayed peak may be possible with fungal infections [32]. Similar to non-neutropenic patients, serial measurement of procalcitonin may be useful in determining the duration of therapy. On the other hand, in a recent study in febrile neutropenic patients undergoing HSCT, procalcitonin showed a limited sensitivity of 66% and a specificity of 75% with a cut-off of 0.5 ng/mL [33]. Furthermore, the procalcitonin-guided protocol did not reduce the use of antibiotics in febrile neutropenia in a randomized controlled trial by Lima et al. [34] In summary, procalcitonin needs to be considered as a supplemental tool for diagnosis, but not as a tool to replace proper clinical and microbiological diagnosis or to withhold initiating antibiotics.

There are other biomarkers such as adrenomedullin or TREM 1 (triggering receptor expressed on myeloid cells-1); adrenomedullin was used in community-acquired pneumonia to predict prognosis and TREM-1, to distinguish bacterial pneumonia from nonbacterial pulmonary disease [35]. Similarly to procalcitonin, the complexity of immunology and the influence of concurrent immunosuppressive medications in the immunocompromised hosts need to be considered when attempting to use these biomarkers.

Rapid Diagnostics

Early identification of bacterial, viral and fungal pathogens and their antimicrobial susceptibility is critical in managing infectious diseases. ASP should assess rapid diagnostics for test accuracy, turn-around time and the extent to which they can prevent the unnecessary initiation or continuation of antimicrobials [36]. ASP should also provide education to providers on the appropriate test population, adequate interpretation of results, limitations of the test, and optimal selection of antimicrobials based on the results [37]. Notably, the benefits of rapid diagnostics will be lost in the absence of real-time ASP interventions [38].

Novel Approaches to Rapid Phenotypic Antimicrobial Susceptibility Testing

Rapid identification of carbapenemase producing Enterobacteriaceaes (CPE) is critical for medical management of this MDR infection as well as for infection control. Rapid Carb Blue Kit (Rosco Diagnostica, Taastrup, Denmark) and Rapidec Carba NP test (bioMerieux, Marcy L'Etoile, France) both detect carbapenemases distinctively from other beta-lactam hydrolyzing enzymes such as ESBL or AmpC (chromosomally encoded or plasmid-mediated) within 2 h. These tests measure color changes caused by carbapenemases-induced imipenem hydrolysis and subsequent acidification of the indicator solution. Both tests have high sensitivity (94–96%) and specificity (96–100%) for carbapenemases including KPC, NDM, VIM and OXA-48 with decreased sensitivity to OXA-48 (94%) [39–41].

Commercially available systems to report identification and susceptibility for the entire antibiogram include the Accelerate PhenoTest BC (Accelerate Diagnostics, Tucson, USA). It uses fluorescence in situ hybridization (FISH) for species identification (1.4 h) and automated time-lapse imaging for susceptibility (6.6 h) directly from positive blood culture [42]. Sensitivity and specificity are 97.5% and 99.3% for identification and 96.3% and 96.4% for susceptibility, respectively. While it provides faster results by approximately 24 h for identification and 42 h for susceptibility with high sensitivity and specificity as compared to standard methods, clinical evidence for patient outcome is lacking. ASP should develop an action plan per test results taking into account the test limitations (eg., false negative identification, major error in susceptibility) to reduce adverse outcomes.

Matrix-Assisted Laser Desorption/Ionization Time-of-Flight Mass Spectrometry (MALDI-TOF MS)

MALDI-TOF MS fingerprinting enables clinical microbiology laboratories to rapidly identify cultured microorganisms. Compared to other biochemical conventional techniques, turnaround times are typically reduced by at least a working day to several days for slower growing species [43]. Vitek MS (BioMerieux, St. Louis, MO, USA) uses MALDI-TOF MS technology to rapidly identify bacteria, viruses and fungi including *Mycobacteria, Nocardia* and molds from different sample origins (e.g., blood, tissue, etc.). Perez *et al*, in their study to include Gram-negative rod bacteremia with ESBL or MDR, found a significant reduction in time to optimal antibiotic therapy (80.9 h v. 23.3 h, $p < 0.001$) and reduced mortality in the intervention group when they adopted MALDI-TOF MS directly from positive blood culture and simultaneously set up for rapid antimicrobial susceptibility testing [44]. Use of MALDI-TOF MS was a significant predictor of survival as well (OR 0.3, 95% confidence interval 0.12–0.79).

Direct Pathogen Identification Using Nucleic Acid Amplification

One example of singleplex PCR as an ASP tool is to adopt nasal MRSA screening to rule out MRSA pneumonia [45]. In a recent meta-analysis by Parente *et al*, nasal MRSA screening showed a high specificity and a negative predictive value (NPV) in ruling out MRSA pneumonia; the NPV was 98.1% for community-acquired MRSA pneumonia and 94.8% for ventilator-associated pneumonia. While current IDSA guidelines for HAP/VAP advocates for empiric MRSA coverage in the presence of a risk factor for MRSA infection [46], many patients can avoid MRSA coverage based on the negative nasal MRSA screening result. Another example is singleplex *C. difficile* PCR. Since *C. difficile* represents the most common cause of infectious diarrhea, *C. difficile* PCR testing should be done prior to ordering the multiplex gastrointestinal panel. One caveat is that the sole use of *C. difficile* PCR is no longer recommended to diagnose *C. difficile* infection due to the extremely high sensitivity of this test and is now to be combined with stool toxin tests [47].

Examples of multiplex PCR include respiratory or meningitis/encephalitis panels from direct respiratory or CSF samples. Interestingly, when using multiplex respiratory virus panels, Semret *et al* found antibiotic management was most significantly associated with radiographic suspicion of pneumonia and less with the RVP results [48]. In other words, other than influenza virus, positivity for viruses was not associated with de-escalation or discontinuation of antibiotics. As highlighted by the authors, when introducing a tool such as a respiratory viral panel, the ability to interpret positive results in the context of the clinical illness and the legitimate concerns of bacterial coinfections need to be addressed.

There are platforms that use nucleic acid amplification for rapid pathogen characterization from positive blood cultures. Examples include Verigene BC (Luminex,

Austin, TX, USA) and FrilmArray BCID (BioMerieux, St. Louis, MO, USA). Some resistant markers are included in the kit and aid in escalation/de-escalation of antibiotics as well.

T2 Candida or T2 Bacteria

Distinguished from other platforms, T2 Candida (T2 Biosystems, Lexington, MA, USA) or T2 Bacteria (T2 Biosystems, Lexington, MA, USA) uses whole blood without the need for culture or nucleic acid extraction [49]. It utilizes PCR amplification from whole blood followed by nanoparticle T2 magnetic resonance detection directly from whole blood allowing detection of candidemia or bacteremia within hours. The rapid turnaround time (i.e., 3–5 h) and high sensitivity- specificity (e.g., 91.1% and 99.4% for T2 Candida) present opportunities for decreased mortality [50]. These tests not only showed enhanced sensitivity as compared to blood cultures, but also offered opportunities for antifungal streamlining based on an excellent specificity. There are clinical data showing decreased time to initiation of antifungals in candidemic patients after adopting the T2 Candida system [51]. Of note, accounting for the imperfect sensitivity of 91.1%, their ASP guideline advocated for empiric antifungal therapy with suspected candidemia in both the pre- and post-T2 candida system [51]. Also, another study by Patch ME *et al* emphasized the importance of paired blood cultures and T2 Candida testing to overcome the imperfect sensitivity of the system. This study showed a decreased time to initiation of antifungal therapy as well as a decreased length of hospital stay by 8 days [52]. ASP should help develop clinical decision support in adopting and interpreting these test results in the appropriate clinical context.

Intravenous to Oral Antibiotics

IV-to-oral conversion is a strategy strongly recommended by the 2016 IDSA guideline [18], and can be safely applied to immunocompromised hosts unless patients cannot tolerate oral therapy or have issues with oral absorption (e.g., significant gastrointestinal (GI) graft-versus-host disease (GVHD), severe mucositis, GI obstruction from tumor). Examples of highly bioavailable antimicrobials that can be switched from IV-to-oral in 1:1 ratio include fluoroquinolones, clindamycin, linezolid, sulfamethoxazole-trimethoprim, metronidazole, and azoles (voriconazole, isavuconazole, fluconazole). When an oral equivalent is not available, infectious diseases consultation can assess and recommend an oral regimen to avoid IV catheters and outpatient parenteral therapy [18].

Antimicrobial Pharmacokinetic and Pharmacodynamics (PK/ PD)

Dose optimization through adequate understanding of antimicrobial PK/PD parameters is another vital stewardship tool. Especially when dealing with MDR organisms leaving limited viable options, maximizing the PK/PD driven dosing for a chosen agent becomes essential. For example, ceftolozane-tazobactam is a broad spectrum anti-pseudomonal cephalosporin whose efficacy is driven by free drug concentration remaining above the minimum inhibitory concentration for a defined proportion of the dosing interval (%*f*T > MIC). It currently has FDA dosing recommendations of 1.5 g q8h given over 1 h for intra-abdominal or urinary tract infection while the clinical trial for hospital-acquired bacterial pneumonia uses a 3 g q8h dosing regimen. In a retrospective review of 35 patients treated with ceftolozane-tazobactam against carbapenem-resistant *P. aeruginosa*, all three patients with a ceftolozane-tazobactam MIC ≥8 mg/L failed therapy and doses used varied between 1.5 and 3 g q8h [53]. On the other hand, when PK/PD was analyzed from a 14 year-old child with cystic fibrosis, %*f*T > MIC for ceftolozane-tazobactam at a MIC of 8 mg/L were 56.3% for 1.5 g q8h (over 1 h) and 93.8% for 3 g q8h (over 3 h), respectively [54]. Furthermore, the human simulated dose of ceftolozane-tazobactam 3 g q8h given over 3 h when combined with amikacin or colistin has shown a synergistic killing effect for *P. aeruginosa* isolates with MICs ≥4 mg/L in an *in vitro* pharmacodynamics model [55]. These findings highlight not only the opportunities for success by maximizing the dose evidenced by PK/PD parameters but also the importance of understanding pharmacodynamic synergy effects between antimicrobials. In the immunocompromised hosts, maximizing PK/PD driven efficacy becomes even more important given the reduced host immune function and the risk of developing resistance due to increased exposure to antimicrobials in this population.

Antimicrobial Allergy Assessment

In the 2016 IDSA and SHEA guidelines for antibiotic stewardship, it is recommended that ASPs promote allergy assessment and penicillin skin testing (PST) when appropriate [18]. Approximately 10% of patients carry a penicillin allergy label [56], and it often impedes the appropriate selection of antibiotics. Antibiotic selection in these patients is associated with inferior microbiological and clinical outcomes (e.g., the less effective use of vancomycin in place of the more effective use of a semisynthetic penicillin for invasive MSSA infection) [57], adverse events (e.g., replacement of penicillin with clindamycin leading to increased *C. difficile* infection), use of more expensive and broader spectrum antibiotics [58], and increased readmissions [59] as well as excess mortality [60]. There are many ASP

Table 1 Antimicrobial stewardship modalities in the immunocompromised hosts

Modalities	Key points
Formulary management	Streamline hospital formulary based on drug interactions, cost, spectrum of coverage, drug supply and usage, dosing, efficacy and safety
Prophylaxis during neutropenia	Provide institutional guidelines for antimicrobial prophylaxis along with international guidelines depending on local patterns of resistance, prior infectious histories, and infectious risks of certain chemotherapy/biologics and cancer diagnosis/ stage
Choice of agents for neutropenic fever	Provide guidelines for the empiric use of anti-MRSA, anti-VRE coverage as well as anti-pseudomonal coverage upon NPF
	Monitor adherence to the guidelines
	Prescreen patients at highest risk for MDR organisms to tailor individualized empiric antibiotics
Early de-escalation after NPF	There are newer data suggesting the feasibility of early de-escalation of anti-pseudomonal beta lactams after NPF
	Until international guidelines are updated reflecting these data, early de-escalation may be attempted in selected patients in consultation with infectious diseases specialists and hematologist/oncologist
Clinical pathway	Interdisciplinary development of local clinical practice guideline is a proven tool to improve implementation
Antimicrobial restriction	Have certain antimicrobials be restricted
	Assess the duration of restricted antimicrobials
Prospective audit and feedback	Allocate necessary resources to identify and prioritize the issues
	Provide persistent effort by dedicated and well-trained personnel
Antifungal stewardship	Antifungal stewardship needs to be in place
	Utilize CT screening, or biomarkers such as Aspergillus galactomannan test for early detection of invasive fungal infection
Use of biomarkers	Kinetics/dynamics of biomarkers can be altered in the immunocompromised hosts, thus requiring careful interpretation when adopted in this population
Rapid diagnostics	Continually evaluate evolving technologies to enhance organism detection, susceptibility and resistance reporting
	Provide clinical decision support involving rapid diagnostics
Intravenous to oral conversion	It can be safely implemented in the immunocompromised hosts unless there are issues with oral absorption such as GI GVHD, GI obstruction from tumor, and severe mucositis
Dose optimization using PK/PD	Maximize antimicrobial efficacy by PK/PD driven dosing when dealing with MDR organisms in the setting of immune deficiency
Allergy assessment	Assess antimicrobial allergy history and record in detail
	Utilize penicillin skin testing if available
	Focus on rashes to differentiate antimicrobial-related rash from other etiologies

NPF neutropenic fever, *CISNE* the clinical index of stable febrile neutropenia, *MRSA* Methicillin-resistant *Staphylococcus aureus*, *VRE* vancomycin-resistant enterococcus, *GI* gastrointestinal, *GVHD* graft-versus-host disease, *PK/PD* pharmacokinetic/dynamic, *MDR* multidrug-resistant

initiatives addressing delabeling of penicillin allergy either combined with PST or not. For example, detailed clinical history by itself has shown to increase delabeling of penicillin allergy [61]. PST driven by Infectious Diseases fellows [62] or pharmacists [63] and resultant delabeling of penicillin allergy have shown significantly increased use of penicillins or cephalosporins in place of broader spectrum, suboptimal or more costly alternative agents. Before concluding a rash was from an antimicrobial, other factors that can cause skin rashes should be considered: namely chemotherapy, GVHD, vasculitis, leukemia cutis, pyoderma gangrenosum, and Sweet's syndrome *et cetera*. In summary, allergy assessment focusing on a detailed characterization of the rash needs to be highlighted in this population along with other basic information such as onset and timing of the reaction, severity, and type of reactions.

Key Points

In the era of antimicrobial resistance, a strong ASP in immunocompromised hosts is of utmost importance for patient safety. There have been many successful practice models embracing ASP strategies in this population (Table 1). There are unique opportunities for ASP in this population including optimal antimicrobial prophylaxis, management of neutropenic fever and early de-escalation after neutropenic fever resolves. Since this population is more vulnerable to opportunistic infections including rare organisms, evolving technologies in rapid diagnostics to enhance sensitivity and the speed of organism detection and susceptibility testing should continually be evaluated and combined with real time ASP interventions when adopted.

References

1. Dellit TH, Owens RC, McGowan JE Jr, et al. Infectious Diseases Society of America and the Society for Healthcare Epidemiology of America Guidelines for Developing an Institutional Program to Enhance Antimicrobial Stewardship. Clin Infect Dis. 2007;44:159–77.
2. Winthrop KL, Mariette X, Silva JT, et al. ESCMID Study Group for Infections in Compromised Hosts (ESGICH) Consensus document on the safety of targeted and biological therapies: an infectious diseases perspective (soluble immune effector molecules [II]: agents targeting interleukins,immunoglobulins and complement factors). Clin Microbiol Infect. 2018;24:S21–40. https://doi.org/10.1016/j.cmi.2018.02.002.
3. So W, Pandya S, Quilitz R, et al. Infectious risks and complications in adult leukemic patients receiving blinatumomab. Mediterr J Hematol Infect Dis. 2018;10(1):e2018029. https://doi.org/10.4084/MJHID.2018.029.

4. National comprehensive cancer network. Prevention and treatment of cancer-related infections version I. 2018. Accessed online on Apr 2018. https://www.nccn.org/professionals/physician_gls/pdf/infections.pdf. Antibiotic prophylaxis for bacterial infections in afebrile neutropenic patients following chemotherapy.
5. Gafter-Gvili A, Fraser A, Paul M, et al. Antibiotic prophylaxis for bacterial infections in afebrile neutropenic patients following chemotherapy. Cochrane Database Syst Rev. 2012;(4):CD004386.
6. Yemm KE, Barreto JN, Mara KC, et al. A comparison of levofloxacin and oral third-generation cephalosporins as antibacterial prophylaxis in acute leukaemia patients during chemotherapy-induced neutropenia. J Antimicrob Chemother. 2018;73:204–11.
7. Taplitz RA, Kennedy EB, Bow EJ, et al. Outpatient management of fever and neutropenia in adults treated for malignancy: American Society of Clinical Oncology and Infectious Diseases Society of America Clinical Practice Guideline Update. J Clin Oncol. 2018:JCO2017776211. https://doi.org/10.1200/JCO.2017.77.6211.
8. Freifeld AG, Bow EJ, Sepkowitz KA, et al. Clinical practice guideline for the use of antimicrobial agents in neutropenic patients with Cancer: 2010 update by the Infectious Diseases Society of America. Clin Infect Dis. 2011;52:e56–93.
9. Tverdek FP, Rolston KV, Chemaly RF. Antimicrobial stewardship in patients with cancer. Pharmacotherapy. 2012;32:722.
10. Giannella M, Bartoletti M, Morelli MC, et al. Risk factors for infection with carbapenem-resistant klebsiella pneumoniae after liver transplantation: the importance of pre and post-transplant colonization. Am J Transplant. 2015;15:1708–15.
11. Lisboa LF, Miranda BG, Vieira MB, et al. Empiric use of linezolid in febrile hematology and hematopoietic stem cell transplantation patients colonized with vancomycin-resistant Enterococcus spp. Int J Infect Dis. 2015;33:171–6.
12. Cho SY, Lee DG, Sm C, et al. Impact of vancomycin resistance on mortality in neutropenic patients with enterococcal bloodstream infection: a retrospective study. BMC Infect Dis. 2013;13:504.
13. Le Clech L, Talarmin JP, Couturier MA, et al. Early discontinuation of empirical antibacterial therapy in febrile neutropenia: the ANTIBIOSTOP study. Infect Dis (Lond). 2018;50(7):539–49. https://doi.org/10.1080/23744235.
14. Averbuch D, Orasch C, Cordonnier C, et al. European guidelines for empirical antibacterial therapy for febrile neutropenic patients in the era of growing resistance: summary of the 2011 4th European conference on infections in leukemia. Haematologica. 2013;98:1826–35.
15. Aguilar-Guisado M, Espigado I, Martin-Pena A, et al. Optimisation of empirical antimicrobial therapy in patients with haematological malignancies and febrile neutropenia (how long study): an open-label, randomized, controlled phase 4 trial. Lancet Haematol. 2017;4:e573–83.
16. Snyder M, Pasikhova Y, Baluch A. Early antimicrobial de-escalation and stewardship in adult hematopoietic stem cell transplantation recipients: retrospective review. Open Forum Infect Dis. 2017;11(4):ofx226. https://doi.org/10.1093/ofid/ofx226.
17. Gustinetti G, Raiola AM, Varaldo R et al. De-escalation and discontinuation of empirical antibiotic treatment in a cohort of allogeneic hematopoietic stem cell transplantation recipients during the pre-engraftment period. Biol Blood Marrow Transplant 2018; pii:S1083-8791(18)30131-9. doi: https://doi.org/10.1016/j.bbmt
18. Barlam TF, Cosgrove SE, Abbo LM, et al. Implementing an antibiotic stewardship program: guidelines by the infectious diseases society of America and the society for healthcare epidemiology of America. Clin Infect Dis. 2016;62:e51.
19. Seo SK, Lo K, Aboo L. Current state of antimicrobial stewardship at solid organ and hematopoietic cell transplant centers in the US. Infect Control Hosp Epidemiol. 2016;37:1195.
20. Metan G, Kaynar L, Yozgat N, et al. A change for the antibacterial treatment policy to decrease carbapenem consumption at a haematopoietic stem cell transplantation centre. Infez Med. 2017;25:33.

21. Nivoix Y, Launoy A, Moulin JC, et al. Adherence to recommendations for the use of antifungal agents in a tertiary care hospital. J Antimicrob Chemother. 2012;67:2506–13.
22. Sutepvarnon A, Apisarnthanarak A, Camins B, et al. Inappropriate use of antifungal medications in a tertiary care center in Thailand: a prospective study. Infect Control Hosp Epidemiol. 2008;29:370–3.
23. Singh N, Wagener MM, Cacciarelli TV, et al. Antifungal management practices in liver transplant recipients. Am J Transplant. 2008;8:426–31.
24. Munoz P, Rojas L, Cervera C, et al. Poor compliance with antifungal drug use guideline by transplant physicians: a framework for educational guidelines and an international consensus on patient safety. Clin Transpl. 2012;26:87–96.
25. Lelievre L, Groh M, Angebault C, et al. Azole resistant Aspergillus fumigates: an emerging problem. Med Mal Infect. 2013;43:139–45.
26. Vallabhaneni S, Cleveland AA, Farley MM, et al. Epidemiology and risk factors for echinocandin nonsusceptible Candida glabrata bloodstream infections: data from a large multisite population-based Candidemia Surveillance Program, 2008-2014. Open Forum Infect Dis. 2015;2:ofv163.
27. Clancy CJ, Nguyen MH. Emergence of Candida auris: an international call to arms. Clin Infect Dis. 2017;64:141–3.
28. Legouge C, Caillot D, Chretien ML, et al. The reversed halo sign: pathognomonic pattern of pulmonary mucormycosis in leukemic patients with neutropenia? Clin Infect Dis. 2014;58:672–8.
29. Millon L, Herbrecht R, Grenouillet F, et al. Early diagnosis and monitoring of mucormycosis by detection of circulating DNA in serum: retrospective analysis of 44 cases collected through the French Surveillance Network of Invasive Fungal Infections (RESSIF). Clin Microbiol Infect. 2016 Sep;22(9):810.e1–8. https://doi.org/10.1016/j.cmi.2015.12.006.
30. Maertens JA, Blennow O, Duarte RF, et al. The current management landscape: aspergillosis. J Antimicrob Chemother. 2016;71(Suppl 2):ii23–9.
31. Brodska H, Drabek T, Malickova K, et al. Marked increase of procalcitonin after the administration of antithymocyte globulin in patients before hematopoietic stem cell transplantation does not indicate sepsis: a prospective study. Crit Care. 2009;13:R37.
32. Sakr Y, Sponholz C, Tuche F, et al. The role of procalcitonin in febrile neutropenic patients: review of the literature. Infection. 2008;36:396–407.
33. Sanchez-Yepes M, Aznar-Oroval E, Lorente-Alegre P, et al. Use of procalcitonin and C-reactive protein in infection markers in febrile neutropenic patients undergoing haematopoietic stem cell transplant. Enferm Infecc Microbiol Clin. 2014;32:418–23.
34. Lima SS, Nobre V, de Castro Romanelli RM et al. Procalcitonin-guided protocol is not useful to manage antibiotic therapy in febrile neutropenia: a randomized controlled trial. Ann Hematol. 2016;95(7):1169–76. https://doi.org/10.1007/s00277-016-2639-5.
35. Stover KR, Kenney RM, King ST, et al. Evaluation of the use of novel biomarkers to augment antimicrobial stewardship program activities. Pharmacotherapy. 2018;38:271–83.
36. Robilotti E, Holubar M, Seo SK, et al. Feasibility and applicability of antimicrobial stewardship in immunocompromised patients. Curr Opin Infect Dis. 2017;30:346–53.
37. Minejima E, Wong-Beringer A. Implementation of rapid diagnostics with antimicrobial stewardship. Expert Rev Anti-Infect Ther. 2016;14:1065–75.
38. Messacar K, Paker SK, Todd JK, et al. Implementation of rapid molecular infectious disease diagnostics: the role of diagnostic and antimicrobial stewardship. J Clin Microbiol. 2017;55:715–23.
39. Novais A, Brilhante M, Pres J, et al. Evaluation of the recently launched rapid carb blue kit for detection of carbapenemase-producing Gram-negative bacteria. J Clin Microbiol. 2015;53:3105–7.
40. Poirel L, Nordmann P. Rapidec carba NP test for rapid detection of carbapenemase producers. J Clin Microbiol. 2015;53:3003–8.

41. Garcia-Fernandez S, Morosini MI, Gijon D, et al. Detection of carbapenemase production in a collection of Enterobacteriaceae with characterized resistance mechanisms from clinical and environmental origins by use of both Carba NP and Blue-Carba tests. J Clin Microbiol. 2016;54:464–6.
42. Lutgring JD, Bittencourt C, TeKippe EM, et al. Evaluation of the accelerate pheno system: result from two academic medical centers. J Clin Microbiol. 2018;56:e01672–17.
43. Cassagne C, Normand AC, L'Ollivier C, et al. Performance of MALDI-TOF MS platforms for fungal identification. Mycoses. 2016;59:678–90.
44. Perez KK, Olsen RJ, Musick WL, et al. Integrating rapid diagnostics and antimicrobial stewardship improves outcomes in patients with antibiotic-resistant Gram-negative bacteremia. J Infect. 2014;69:216–25.
45. Parente DM, Cunha CB, Mylonakis E, et al. The clinical utility of methicillin resistant Staphylococcus aureus (MRSA) nasal screening to rule out MRSA pneumonia: a diagnostic meta-analysis with antimicrobial stewardship implications. Clin Infect Dis. 2018;67:1–7. https://doi.org/10.1093/cid/ciy024.
46. Kalil AC, Metersky ML, Klompas M, et al. Management of adults with hospital-acquired and ventilator-associated pneumonia: 2016 clinical practice guidelines by the Infectious Diseases Society of America and the American Thoracic Society. Clin Infect Dis. 2016;63:e61–111.
47. McDonald LC, Gerding DN, Johnson S, et al. Clinical practice guidelines for Clostridium difficile infection in adults and children: 2017 update by the Infectious Diseases Society of America (IDSA) and Society for Healthcare Epidemiology of America (SHEA). Clin Infect Dis. 2018;xx(00):1–48.
48. Semret M, Schiller I, Jardin BA, et al. Multiplex respiratory virus testing for antimicrobial stewardship: a prospective assessment of antimicrobial use and clinical outcomes among hospitalized adults. J Infect Dis. 2017;216:936–44.
49. Pfaller MA, Wolk DM, Lowery TJ. T2MR and T2Candida: novel technology for the rapid diagnosis of candidemia and invasive candidiasis. Future Micoribiol. 2016;11:103–17.
50. Mylonakis E, Clancy CJ, Ostrosky-Zeichner L, et al. T2 magnetic resonance assay for the rapid diagnosis of candidemia in whole blood: a clinical trial. Clin Infect Dis. 2015;60:892–9.
51. Wilson JM, Alangaden G, Tibbetts RJ, et al. T2 magnetic resonance assay improves timely management of candidemia. J Antimicrob Stewardship. 2017;1:12–8.
52. Patch ME, Weisz E, Cubillos A, et al. Impact of rapid, culture-independent diagnosis of candidaemia and invasive candidiasis in a community health system. J Antimicrob Chemother. 2018;73:iv27–30.
53. Munita JM, Aitken SL, Miller WR, et al. Multicenter evaluation of ceftolozane/tazobactam for serious infections caused by carbapenem-resistant Pseudomonas aeruginosa. Clin Infect Dis. 2017;65:158–61.
54. Ang JY, Abdel-Haq N, Zhu F, et al. Multidrug-resistant Pseudomonas aeruginosa infection in a child with cystic fibrosis. Antimicrob Agents Chemother. 2016;60:5627–30.
55. Rico-Caballero V, Abuhussain SA, Kuti JL et al. Efficacy of human-simulated exposures of ceftolozane/tazobactam alone and in combination with amikacin or colistin against multidrug-resistant Pseudomonas aeruginosa in an in vitro pharmacodynamics model. Antimicrob Agents Chemother 2018. pii: AAC.02384-17. doi: https://doi.org/10.1128/AAC.02384-17.
56. Trubiano JA, Pai Mangalore R, Baey YW, et al. Old but not forgotten: antibiotic allergies in general medicine (the AGM study). Med J Aust. 2016;204:273.
57. Gonzalez C, Rubio M, Romero-Vivas J, et al. Bacteremic pneumonia due to Staphylococcus aureus: a comparison of disease caused by methicillin-resistant and methicillin-susceptible organisms. Clin Infect Dis. 1999;29:1171.
58. Li M, Krishna MT, Razag S, et al. A real-time prospective evaluation of clinical pharmacoeconomic impact of diagnostic label of 'penicillin allergy' in a UK teaching hospital. J Clin Pathol. 2014;67:1088–92.

59. Blumenthal KG, Shenov ES, Varughese CA, et al. Impact of a clinical guideline for prescribing antibiotics to inpatients reporting penicillin or cephalosporin allergy. Ann Allergy Asthma Immunol. 2015;115:294–300.
60. Charneski L, Deshpande G, Smith SW, et al. Impact of an antimicrobial allergy label in the medical record on clinical outcomes in hospitalized patients. Pharmacotherapy. 2011;31:742–7.
61. Sigona NS, Steele JM, Miller CD. Impact of a pharmacist-driven beta-lactam allergy interview on inpatient antimicrobial therapy: a pilot project. J Am pharm Assoc (2003). 2016;56:665.
62. Heil EL, Bork JT, Schmalzle SA, et al. Implementation of an infectious disease fellow-managed penicillin allergy skin testing service. Open Forum Infect Dis. 2016;3:ofw155.
63. Chen JR, Tarver SA, Alvarez KS, et al. A proactive approach to penicillin allergy testing in hospitalized patients. J Allergy Clin Immunol Pract. 2017;5:686–93.

Index

A. P. Velez et al. (eds.), *Infections in Neutropenic Cancer Patients*,
https://doi.org/10.1007/978-3-030-21859-1

Q

R

S

MIX
Papier aus verantwortungsvollen Quellen
Paper from responsible sources
FSC® C105338

If you have any concerns about our products,
you can contact us on
ProductSafety@springernature.com

In case Publisher is established outside the EU,
the EU authorized representative is:
Springer Nature Customer Service Center GmbH
Europaplatz 3, 69115 Heidelberg, Germany

Printed by Libri Plureos GmbH
in Hamburg, Germany